Understanding Depression

PROFESSOR ASHOKA JAHNAVI PRASAD

All Rights Reserved

This book contains material protected under International and Federal Copyright Laws and Treaties. This e-book is intended for personal use only. Any unauthorized reprint or use of this material is prohibited. No part of this book may be used in any commercial manner without express permission of the author. Scholarly use of quotations must have proper attribution to the published work. This work may not be deconstructed, reverse engineered or reproduced in any other format.

To my patients

Table of Contents

PREFACE

Part One

1. THE BASIC QUESTIONS AND THE PSYCHOLOGICAL APPROACH

2. CRITICAL REVIEW OF THE MAJOR CONCEPTS OF DEPRESSION

3. THE MANIFEST SYMPTOMATOLOGY OF DEPRESSION IN ADULTS

4. MANIFEST SYMPTOMATOLOGY OF DEPRESSION IN CHILDREN AND ADOLESCENTS

Part Two

5. THE PSYCHOBIOLOGY OF SADNESS

6. PSYCHODYNAMICS OF SEVERE DEPRESSION

7. PSYCHODYNAMICS OF MILD DEPRESSION

8. PSYCHODYNAMICS OF DEPRESSION AND SUICIDE IN CHILDREN AND ADOLESCENTS

Part Three

9. PSYCHOTHERAPY OF SEVERE DEPRESSION

10. PSYCHOTHERAPY OF SEVERE DEPRESSION: CASE REPORTS

11. POSTPARTUM DEPRESSION

12. PSYCHOTHERAPY OF DEPRESSION DURING THE MIDDLE YEARS (INVOLUTIONAL MELANCHOLIA)

13. PSYCHOTHERAPY OF MILD DEPRESSION

14. CASE ILLUSTRATION: THE PSYCHOTHERAPY OF MILD DEPRESSION

15. PSYCHOTHERAPY OF DEPRESSION IN CHILDREN AND ADOLESCENTS

Part Four

16. PART ONE: SOCIOCULTURAL FACTORS, SOCIOLOGY OF KNOWLEDGE, AND DEPRESSION

    PART TWO: DEPRESSION AND METHODS OF CHILD-REARING

17. FRANZ KAFKA: A LITERARY PROTOTYPE

OF THE DEPRESSIVE CHARACTER

Part Five

18. ADDITIONAL REMARKS ON THE RELATION BETWEEN COGNITION AND DEPRESSION

REFERENCES

PREFACE

The abnormal state of the psyche called depression has been known since biblical and Homeric times, but the present decade has seen an unusual intensification of interest in this disorder. The condition is very common and affects many people in various degrees, ranging from relatively mild disturbances to the most severe types of suffering.

Recent interest has focused on the study of depression as a metabolic disorder, to be treated exclusively or predominantly with drug therapy. This book is the effort of many clinicians who belong to what is today a minority, but a vocal minority which wants to be heard as widely as possible, for its exponents feel they have important things to say, even to psychiatrists who follow a basically different approach.

With the present work, we wish to illustrate the importance of psychological factors in both the etiology and the therapy of depression. We attempt to clarify how these factors came to be and how their effects can be corrected or resolved. These psychological factors may not be the only ones involved in every case of depression, but we believe they are necessary;

they are always there to be found if we know how to search for them, and we must account for them, unless we settle for a superficial and symptomatic recovery which may relapse at any time. Even a therapist who treats depressed patients mainly with tricyclics and monoamine oxidase (MAO) inhibitors cannot help practicing some kind of psychotherapy, cannot help inquiring about the dynamics of the patient's anguish and conflict, cannot refrain from interpreting the patient's past history and what goes on in the therapeutic situation.

After reviewing the major theories of depression and describing the clinical symptomatology of its various forms, we examine the psychodynamics and psychotherapy of this condition in adults, children, and adolescents. Special chapters are devoted to the depressions occurring postpartum and in the middle years. One of the early chapters deals with the psychobiology of sadness—a knowledge of which is a prerequisite to the understanding of depression. One of the last chapters deals with the sociocultural factors which may be intimately involved in the engendering of depression.

The field of depression is vast, and no single psychiatrist can master it in its entirety. Each of us has written the sections of the book that deal with the areas of his respective competence. One of my colleagues prepared the chapters on severe depressions in adults, as well as one on the questions of the psychological approach: chapters 1, 3, 5, 6, 9, 10, 11, and 12. Another prepared the chapters on mild depression in adults and those on depression in children and adolescents, as well as a chapter on the major concepts of depression: chapters 2, 4, 7,8,13,14,15,17, and 18. Chapter 16, which deals with sociocultural factors, is divided into two parts.

Although I conceived this work in its general content, policy, and major points of view, no page of the book has been written in collaboration. In each chapter the respective author is indicated.

We hope that the detailed case reports presented in chapters 10, 11, 12, and 14 will illustrate at a practical level the nature of our work and will clarify the theoretical premises reported in other chapters.

Those who look for confirmation from statistics gathered from studying large numbers of patients will not find what they seek in this book. This statistical type of study is incompatible with an in-depth and thorough psychodynamic investigation which limits the number of individuals who can be studied. Although we feel that we have covered a vast panorama of depression from childhood to maturity, depth has been our prime concern and not the number of patients treated.

If the reading of this book succeeds in convincing our colleagues that this approach is effective and not at all difficult to follow once the therapist has overcome his first hesitations and reservations, we shall feel fulfilled in our effort. We shall renew our hopes that many others will pursue and further explore this promising type of research and therapy.

Professor Ashoka

Jahnavi Prasad

PART ONE

Basic Notions and Manifest Symptomatology

[1]

THE BASIC QUESTIONS AND THE PSYCHOLOGICAL APPROACH

Silvano Arieti

Common is the sorrow that visits the human being when an adverse event hits his precarious existence or when the discrepancy between the way life is and the way it possibly could be becomes the center of his fervid reflection. In some people this sorrow comes and goes repeatedly, and in some others, only from time to time. It is painful, delays actions, and generally heals, often but not always after deepening its host's understanding and hastening his maturation.

Less common—but frequent enough to constitute a major psychiatric concern—is the sorrow that does not abate with the passage of time, that seems exaggerated in relation to the supposed precipitating event, or inappropriate, or unrelated to any discernible cause, or replacing a more congruous emotion. This sorrow slows down, interrupts, or disrupts one's actions; it spreads a sense of anguish which may become difficult to contain; at times it tends to expand relentlessly into a psyche which seems endless in its capacity to experience mental pain; often it recurs even after appearing to be healed. This emotional state is generally called depression.

Is it just a feeling? Is it a syndrome? Is it a disease? It is a feeling but, contrary to common sorrow and sadness, it is also a syndrome insofar as it brings about severe alterations of psychological and some somatic functions. Whether or not it is a disease depends on the definition given to the term disease. If "disease" means a condition that causes a dysfunction of the organism, irrespective of evidence of cellular pathology and irrespective of the nature of the cause which determined it, we can certainly call depression a disease. Again, we must carefully differentiate depression from sadness and normal sorrow, which is a topic we shall take into consideration in chapter 5. Depression thus implies deviation from the normal way of experiencing some emotions, including sadness and sorrow.

One of the basic and most frequently asked questions is whether this deviation from the normal is *dependent upon external circumstances.* Many authors have emphatically stressed that depression is not dependent upon external circumstances; at times a dependency seems to exist, but it is illusory. An unpleasant event which would elicit only temporary sadness or sorrow in the normal person, brings about in the patient a psychiatric illness that soon reveals an autonomous process. This psychiatric illness is at first difficult to distinguish from normal sadness, but eventually it is accompanied by agitation and restlessness or by severe retardation, inhibition, reduction in responsiveness to external stimuli, and recurrent sequences of gloomy and pessimistic thoughts. In some cases —those labeled manic-depressive— this psychiatric picture alternates with periods of euphoria and motor excitement.

If this condition is an illness or a medical entity, and if it is not found to be connected with external circumstances and has an autonomous development, then the conclusion drawn by many is that it is an endogenous condition; that is, originating within the organism itself.

When such a position is taken, research along certain lines of inquiry receives momentum. Inasmuch as neuropathological research proved to be completely useless since the time of Kraepelin (1921), the major fields investigated have been the genetic and the biochemical. It is not within the scope of this book to cover these two vast fields. We shall mention only that several authors have found evidence that at least in biphasic manicdepressive psychosis (a disorder characterized by both depressive and manic attacks) there is a genetic factor. (See Mendels, 1974; Cadoret and Tanna, 1977.) Perris (1966) also reached the conclusion that patients who suffer from both manic and depressive episodes are to be genetically distinguished from those who suffer only from depressive attacks. In a subsequent article, Perris (1976) reached the moderate conclusion that "the combined results of clinical and biological studies of affective disorders support the hypothesis that genetic factors are of some importance for the occurrence of at least some groups of these disorders" (especially those presenting both the manic and the depressive phases).

Contrasting with quite a large number of authors who have concluded that a genetic factor may be involved in the typical biphasic manic depressive disorder is the work of Odegard (1963), which showed no genetic difference between psychotic and neurotic forms of depression. In summary, a genetic factor seems to have been almost convincingly demonstrated only in typical cases of manic-depressive psychosis. In them, too, however, it seems to be in the nature of a predisposition, and not a factor sufficient in itself to bring about the clinical condition.

If studies on heredity are far from conclusive, biochemical studies are even more so. The most promising line of research has followed the catecholamine hypothesis, according to which depression may be connected with decreased activity of some amine synaptic neurotransmitters, probably norepinephrine and dopamine. Conversely, in manic states there would be increased activity of these amines. This hypothesis and others have not gone beyond the hypothetical stage. (See Mendels, Stern, and Frazer, 1976.)

Another issue which to my knowledge has not been investigated is that the biological predisposition may consist of a greater facility to activate specific neuronal spatio-temporal patterns in the brain. These spatio-temporal patterns ultimately would engage more intensively than usual those parts of the limbic system or other parts of the brain that mediate the phenomenon of depression.

I am not in a position to say whether these altered patterns ultimately could be subsumed in the category of altered biochemical events. But it seems to me that we should not bypass in a cavalier fashion a level of investigation which has been followed in the studies of other functions— for instance, language. Obviously we cannot believe that there is a center of sadness and depression which is similar to language centers or even to the pleasure center that the experiments by Olds and Milner (1954) suggest. If areas which mediate sadness and depression do exist, they probably consist of many cerebral areas, not contiguous, but working together through neuronal associations and constituting what Luria (1966, 1.973) called a functional system.

In contrast with my hesitation in taking any position about the previous matter is the security with which I can make the following affirmation: in the several decades spent in psychiatric practice and research, I have never treated for a considerable length of time a case of depression about which I could say that there was no psychological factor involved. I have never seen a patient about whom I could say that his depression was unrelated to a prior anguish, or about whom I could say that his depression came from nowhere and its origin had to be sought exclusively in a metabolic disorder. And yet I want to stress that my experience deals predominantly with cases of severe depression that many authors call endogenous. Bemporad (who is not the author of this chapter), joins me in asserting that in the mild cases of depression which he has treated there was always some psychological factor involved.

Does this mean that the position taken in this book is that every case of depression is a *reactive* depression? Not at all, at least in the sense in which the word reaction is used by many psychiatrists. The concept of psychiatric illness as a reaction is attributed by some to Karl Bonhoeffer, who described what he called

"exogenous reactions" (1910). However, Bonhoeffer referred to diseases of the brain caused by external toxic agents. He interpreted mental illness as a reaction to a physical alteration.

In the United States the concept of depression as a reaction derives from the works and teachings of Adolph Meyer. Although Meyer was much more interested in schizophrenia, he also enunciated for depression some principles that followed his general psychiatric orientation. He spoke of patients who "are apt to *react* with a peculiar depressive reaction where others get along with fair balance" (1908a). (Italics mine.) In the same article Meyer stated, .. the etiology thus involves (1) constitutional make-up and (2) a precipitating factor; and in our eagerness we cut out the latter and only speak of the heredity or constitutional make-up. It is my contention that we must use *both* facts and that of the two, for *prevention* and for special characterization of the make-up, the precipitating factor is of the greater importance because it alone gives us an idea of the actual defect and a suggestion as to how to strengthen the person that he may become resistive." (Italics in the original.)

Adolph Meyer's words, written in 1908, retain their poignancy today. Meyer stressed that both factors have to be considered. He italicized "both" but not "reaction." Although Meyer referred to the precipitating factor as being important "because it alone gives us an idea of the actual defect," American psychiatry subsequently gave the emphasis to the concept of reaction. But what was the nature of the defect to which Meyer referred? We know from his other works and especially from his studies on schizophrenia that he felt both the "actual defect" and the reaction were the result of the total life experience of the patient as well as of his biological endowment (the psychobiologic set). However, if Meyer was not able to penetrate sufficiently into the depth psychology of the schizophrenic, even though he studied him longitudinally, he was even less able to do so with the depressed patient. Although Meyer very correctly stressed that "the reaction" would not occur in psychiatric patients if they had not been prepared for it, he investigated this preparation in a vague and unsatisfactory way; namely as "substitutive activity" (Meyer, 1908*b*). As a result of Meyer's influence, American psychiatrists could be divided into two groups: the group who gave importance only to the reaction and saw the patient as a passive entity dominated by the external event; and the group who retained the old conception that the patient was suffering from an endogenous disease and therefore was to be viewed as an organism at the mercy of its chromosomic or metabolic destiny.

It is not the aim of this book to demonstrate or deny the existence of constitutional or biochemical factors. Whether such factors exist is not of major relevance to our theme, according to which other factors— psychological factors— must exist or at least coexist. Inasmuch as every psychological event requires neurophysiological and biochemical mechanism for its occurrence, in this book the existence of such mechanisms is reaffirmed but not studied.

Although the authors of this book give major importance to psychological factors, they do not subscribe to the usual concept of reaction. When the authors use the word "reaction" to describe some forms of depression in which the precipitating event seems of major importance (for instance, in the so-called reactive depression), they follow a commonly adopted terminology in order to prevent possible confusion.

The reason that does not permit us to embrace the concept of reaction, even in cases where the precipitating event exists and is likely to be of the greatest importance, is the conclusion drawn from our studies that such an event would not have become a precipitating factor unless it had a special meaning for the patient, and consequently an assumed pathogenetic power. Thus the environment and the patient both contribute to the transformation of the event into a cause: the environment, by offering the contingency of the event; the patient,

by attributing either consciously or unconsciously a special meaning to the event. Furthermore, the event would not be given such a meaning and would not be endowed with such power if the patient had not integrated his past life experiences and personality in specific ways.

For many years I have indicated (and Bemporad, through clinical work, has also confirmed) that a preceding ideology prepares the ground for depression. The ideology is responsible for the special meaning given to the precipitating event and for the way the patient deals with that event. When there is no recognizable precipitating event, there is nevertheless a special preexisting ideology which to some extent consciously, and to a much larger extent unconsciously, has prepared the ground for the depressive outcome. The ideology, which had an integrative function in the life of the patient and was used as a defense, now makes him experience a state of partial or total loss, helplessness, or hopelessness which is accompanied by depression. Whereas the depression generally remains as a subjective and

conscious phenomenon, the cognitive substratum may become partially or totally unconscious.

In this book we shall illustrate how this ideology came to be. In many cases its origin can be traced to childhood events. However, it will be apparent to the reader that although we consider childhood experiences very important, in agreement with classic Freudian tenets, we do not consider them the exclusive determinants of a psychopathological course of events as it unfolds in the life history of the patient.

In the terminology of general systems theory, the psyche is not a closed system but a system open to continuous influences from factors occurring outside the system (Bertalanffy, 1956). Psychopathological structures are also open systems. They are states of various degrees of improbability that are maintained by negative psychological entropy coming from outside the original system. An open system such as the psyche follows the principle of equifinality; the final state is not unequivocally determined by the initial condition. Each stage of life is under the influence of the previous stages, but not in rigid or ineluctable ways. Other factors intervene. Early experiences participate in causing depression only when, together with other factors, they facilitate the formation of an ideology which will lead to unfavorable patterns of living.

Several issues emerge from the foregoing. Even though we speak of patterns of living and of specific behavior throughout this book, we do not focus on the external behavior, but on the ideology and subsequent mechanisms that lead to the formation of these patterns. It is for this reason that our approach is called cognitive. Although I have done psychiatric research on cognition since 1946, my first writings on cognition in reference to depression appeared in 1959 and 1962. Since 1963 Aaron Beck has also stressed the cognitive approach to depression. The approach that I have proposed and to which Bemporad has added a number of original contributions differs from Beck's in that our approach is longitudinal and dynamic. It does not stress the point that the patient is depressed because he has depressive thoughts, but it puts in evidence a cognitive history whose existence was to a considerable extent unconscious. Many people experience reluctance to accept a cognitive approach lest the affective life and especially motivation, conscious and unconscious, be disregarded or not recognized in its full role. This apprehension particularly is felt in connection with the study and treatment of affective disorders, in which the major deviation from the normal involves affects.

A prevailing cultural anti-intellectualism has caused misapprehensions and distortions even in the fields of psychiatry and psychoanalysis. A cognitive approach stresses a fact which is very seldom acknowledged in psychiatry and psychoanalysis: at a human level most emotions do not exist without a cognitive substratum. The expansion of the neocortex and consequently of our cognitive functions also has permitted an expansion of our affective life. In a classic paper published in 1937, Papez demonstrated that several parts of the rhinencephalon and archipallium (included now after MacLean, 1959, in the limbic system) are not used for olfactory functions in the human being, but for experiencing emotion. In spite of the diminished importance of olfaction, these areas have expanded rather than decreased in man, and have become associated with vast neocortical areas. Elsewhere (Arieti, 1967) I have shown that in the human being elementary emotions, which can exist without or with relatively little cognitive counterpart—such as tension, fear, and rage—are changed into higher emotions (anxiety, anger, depression, hate, and so forth) through the intervention of complicated cognitive mechanisms. It is because of these connections with a potentially infinite realm of symbolic cognition that the emotional life of the human being also becomes immense and potentially infinite. In chapter 5 I shall illustrate how cognitive elements can give rise to sadness and depression.

At the beginning of this century, Bleuler and Jung introduced into psychiatry the concept of "complex." According to Laplanche and Pontalis (1973) a complex is an "organized group of ideas and memories of great affective force which are either partly or totally unconscious. Complexes are constituted on the basis of the interpersonal relationships of childhood history; they may serve to structure all levels of the psyche: emotions, attitudes, adapted behavior."

The concept of complex was embraced immediately by classic psychoanalysts, but Freud soon found it to be an unsatisfactory theoretical notion (Jones, 1955). Since then it has lost popularity in psychoanalytic and psychiatric circles, although gaining great popularity in common parlance. A complex is referred to in this book as a cognitive construct or as a system of constructs. The old term "complex" has lost value in professional circles because not enough importance was given to its cognitive components. It is understood that when we refer to a construct we do not connote something static, but something potentially capable of changing throughout the life of the individual; something which is altered by life events and at the same time is a promoter of other life events.

Although it is important to study the transformation from the cognitive to the affective components of the psyche, it is equally important to study why in our psychiatric cases it is so difficult for the patient to free himself from the intense feeling of depression. Often he cannot escape from the feeling of having lost what was most valuable to him, either something specific or something very vague, undefinable, or impossible to express with words. In serious cases the patient mourns the most profound loss, the loss of life's meaning—an experience which reflects in magnified form an original loss or a series of factual or symbolic losses. In these very serious cases the patient feels or acts as if he had reached an inevitable conclusion that his life is meaningless and worthless. The intense depression that accompanies this apparent conclusion actually betrays the patient's attachment to and love for life, and his inherent premise that life is meaningful and should be worthwhile. There is thus something psychologically positive even in this deep depression. In his inner self the patient is not one of those people who consider the events of the cosmos to be due to random collisions of atoms, transformed by chance into organized unities, and completely independent from the needs of the human heart.

Outside the realm of pathology, is there anything similar to this deep depression which implies the inevitability of what is dreaded most? Yes: the *tragic* situation. The relation between depression and tragedy will be studied in chapter 16.

Before proceeding to discuss further the cognitive approach, I must mention that the other psychological interpretations of depression are reviewed by Bemporad in chapter 2. In chapter 16 the relation between depression and some ideologies to which the patient is exposed in his sociocultural environment also are described and discussed.

The major themes of this book will be, however, the psychopathology and psychotherapy of the individual patient—child, adolescent, and adult. When we go beyond the study of manifest symptomatology and make our first acquaintance with the history of the depressed patient, we feel as if an invisible force, running throughout his life, has brought him to his present predicament. One of the main aims of this book is to make visible that invisible force, by showing how it came into existence and sustained itself on many facts, internal and external, individual and sociocultural; most of them unconscious and others conscious, but with unconscious ramifications.

Another purpose of this book is to illustrate

in detail our psychotherapeutic approach. The psychotherapist intends to affect the psychological etiological factors and mechanisms to such an extent that even when biological mechanisms enter into the picture, by themselves they will not be able to maintain the disorder, at least with the same degree of intensity. A successful psychotherapy also will make much less likely the recurrence of the disorder. We hope that our case reports will support our optimism. We have come to the conclusion that most cases of depression, ranging from mild to severe, benefit from psychotherapy. We do not object to the use of other types of treatment in some cases, but we feel that for many patients the psychotherapeutic approach will prove very rewarding, even when other types of therapy have failed. Combined forms of treatment also can be used in a few selected cases.

Although the patient is by far our major concern, we should not omit considering that the psychotherapeutic approach also is rewarding for the therapist, who learns in greater depth some dimensions of human existence. As I wrote elsewhere (1976), when we successfully treat a patient who has been severely depressed we experience a burst of joy because we have helped a person who is happy to have known us. But we also feel a secret joy because we have come to know the patient, and in knowing him we know more of ourselves. There is always a resonance in our heart for the anguish of the depressed which does not seem to us completely unfounded, but similar to ours, and containing a partial truth based on the human predicament.

This study of the depressed person will show how we ourselves can contribute to our own sorrow with the strange ways in which we mix and give meaning to our ideas and feelings. We shall learn that the study of life circumstances is important, but that even more important is the study of our ideas about these circumstances, our ideals and what we do with them, and how we use them to create feelings. This study will explore, and we hope to some extent enlighten, not just our pathology but our so-called normality; not just our despair but our confident expectation; not just our loneliness but also our ways of helping each other and reinforcing the human bond.

[2]

CRITICAL REVIEW OF THE MAJOR CONCEPTS OF DEPRESSION

Jules Bemporad

> Melancholia is one of the great words of psychiatry. Suffering many mutations, at one time the guardian of outworn schemes or errant theories, presently misused, cavilled at, dispossessed, it has endured into our own times, a part of medical terminology no less than of common sense.
>
> *Sir Aubrey Lewis*

Introduction

Depression, perhaps unlike any other disorder in psychiatry or in medicine in general, traces its history to the first written records of mankind. Various characters of ancient myths or protagonists in the Bible are depicted as manifesting symptoms which today would be classified as typical of depressive illness. The first objective clinical description of depression was made by Hippocrates, who coined the term "melancholia," intending to call attention to the surfeit of black bile in the depressed individual.

The significance of the early records, as noted by Zilboorg (1944), is that they demonstrate that the symptoms of affective illness have remained essentially the same for twenty-five centuries. Despite this historical consistency of symptom description, the proposed causes and treatments of depression have been revised consistently, reflecting the etiological and theoretical fashions of the day. Therefore any comprehensive summary of the history of depression amounts to a documentation of the evolution of psychiatric thought. In consideration of this enormous literature, I will discuss only those authors who were either pioneers in advancing novel ideas on depression or whose thoughts on depression continue to exert a considerable influence on current conceptualizations.[1]

The Delineation of a Syndrome

Hippocrates, who is said to have lived in the fourth century BC, gave the first medical description of depression, which he called melancholia, believing it to be caused by an excess of black bile in the brain. He concluded that melancholia was closely related to epilepsy and categorized it with mania, phrenitis, and paranoia as one of the four major types of psychiatric illness. Although Hippocrates may claim priority as the first to describe the disorder, it was Aretaeus of Cappadocia who in the second century AD wrote the most complete, and remarkably modern, depiction of depression. Aretaeus proposed that depression was caused by purely psychological factors and it had little to do with either bile, phlegm, or humours. Aretaeus also seems to have antedated Kraepelin by seventeen centuries in associating mania with depression in certain cases and by considering both conditions as part of a single disease entity. He may even have given a more accurate prognosis than Kraepelin, noting that the illness recurred despite remissions, and recovery from one episode did not ensure cure (Arieti, 1974). Finally, Aretaeus appreciated the significance of interpersonal relationships in the course of depression, reporting the case of a severely disturbed patient who recovered when he fell in love.

We may further appreciate his contributions in the description below, which is remarkably similar to our own contemporary textbooks:

"The characteristic appearances, then, are not obscure; for the patients are dull or stern, dejected or unreasonably torpid, without any manifest cause: such is the commencement of melancholy. And they also become peevish, dispirited, sleepless and start up from a disturbed sleep .... They are prone to change their minds readily; to become bossy, meanspirited, illiberal, and in a little time, perhaps, simple, extravagant, munificent, not from any virtue of soul, but from the changeableness of the disease. But if the illness becomes more urgent, hatred, avoidance of the haunts of men, vain lamentations are seen; they complain of life and desire to die." (Quoted in Lewis, 1934.)

This promising work on depression initiated by Aretaeus (and also by Celsus, who wrote insightful descriptions of depression) was unfortunately not continued by his immediate successors. Galen in the second century also developed a theory of mental illness based on alleged humours. His theory remained doctrine throughout the Middle Ages. It was not until the Renaissance that a renewed interest in depression and an original approach to its causes appeared. This was especially true in Elizabethan England, where an apparent epidemic of melancholia seems to have occurred, as evident from the number of works devoted to this disorder in that short period of history. Timothy Bright published his *Treatise on Melancholia* in 1586 and twenty years later Thomas

Walkington's *Optick Glass of Humours* appeared, which dealt extensively with the "melancholick complexion" resulting from humours and the effect of the planets (Veith, 1970). Finally, in 1621 Robert Burton finished his massive *Anatomy of Melancholy* which is still available today. This immense, meandering work is as much a reflection on life as a tome on depression. Despite its encyclopedic comprehensiveness and erudition, it is difficult to distill a central theme on depression in terms of either cause or treatment. Physicians on the continent were discovering again that melancholia and mania often alternate in the same individuals. Bonet in 1684, Schact in 1747, and Herchel in 1768 all associated the two conditions as part of one diagnostic entity.

With the spread of the scientific revolution, psychiatric investigators began to look upon mental illness as caused physiologically rather than by demonic possession. However, there was little overall order in their discoveries; each investigator claimed to have found a new syndrome on the basis of a few patients. It was a time of extremely detailed delineation of pathological states, sanctified by Latin terminology for each diagnostic entity. Falret in

1851 differentiated between ordinary melancholia and the episodic variety, and three years later Baillarger made a similar observation. Falret also coined the term "folie circulaire" and described in some patients the occurrence of healthy intervals, which contrasted with gradual but definite degeneration in other individuals. Falret's other significant contributions were his observations that recurrent depression seemed to be familial and females were more frequently affected. However, the state of the art was actually one of confusion; there was little correspondence between the diagnostic divisions made by different psychiatrists. One general theme that did emerge was the preoccupation with the outcome of a disorder, which then was used to certify its diagnosis. Greisinger in the midnineteenth century divided "insanity" into two broad categories: recoverable and incurable. Perhaps the interest in prognosis resulted from a lack of suitable treatment methods, so that studying the course of an illness and then classifying it was the best that could be done.

This state of affairs may help to explain the tremendous contribution of Kraepelin, who revolutionized psychiatry by establishing a nosological system that continues to be used today. Kraepelin sifted out the common elements from the confusion of individualistic syndromes and consolidated these into three major categories of illness: dementia praecox, paraphrenia, and manic-depressive psychosis. He based his classifications on both the similarity of symptoms and the eventual outcome of the disorder.

Kraepelin included a variety of depressive disorders under the larger category of manicdepressive psychosis. He reasoned that this group of disorders shared common symptoms despite superficial differences, that different symptoms might replace one another in the same patient, and that there was a uniformly benign prognosis (Arieti, 1974). In Kraepelin's nosological system, the following mental states were included under manic-depressive psychosis: intermittent psychosis, simple mania, some cases of confusion, most cases of melancholia, and certain cases of mild mood disorders that were prodromal of a more severe condition. Overall, he distinguished four major subgroups: depressive states, manic states, mixed states, and fundamental states, that is, disorders of mood experienced between, before, or as replacing manic-depressive attacks (Braceland, 1957).

Kraepelin's great contribution to psychiatry was in imposing order on the nosological chaos that had existed before him. According to Braceland (1957), when Kraepelin entered psychiatry "workers were floundering helplessly around in a morass of symptoms for which they were unable to find any common denominators" (p. 872). In his attempt at a workable system of classification, Kraepelin followed the medical model; he viewed psychiatric disorders as having an (as yet) unidentified but certain organic cause, a characteristic course, and a predictable outcome.

In keeping with this set of criteria, he differentiated manic-depressive psychosis from dementia praecox, in that the former condition was remitting and normal health returned despite severe derangement during clinical episodes. In a sense Kraepelin created a psychiatry of end results, utilizing prognosis as a major diagnostic criterion.

Although Kraepelin's system was widely adopted and hailed as a major progressive step, it also had its critics. It was argued that in view of the great number of influences (from without and within) acting on any individual, a strictly deterministic prognosis could not be maintained with certainty. In his later writings, Kraepelin conceded the validity of this criticism and admitted that a certain percentage of cases did not follow the prescribed course. However, Kraepelin's critics were not so much concerned with his clinical data as with his fatalistic view of illness and his use of outcome (which could not be known for a single patient) in making a diagnosis.

One of Kraepelin's most vocal critics was Adolf Meyer, whose own system of classification in contrast was based on a broader category of reaction types. Meyer had initially welcomed and employed the new Kraepelinian system but he eventually grew skeptical of it because it relied too heavily on outcome. Meyer began to treat psychiatric disorders as influenced by life events rather than by strictly organic conditions that progress regardless of environmental factors. Meyer eventually discarded the disease model entirely, preferring to view psychiatric disorders as an individual's specific reactions to a succession of life events. In 1904 Meyer argued against the term melancholia, stating that it gave a stamp of certainty to a vague condition of which little sure knowledge existed. He suggested that the disorder be called depression, at least until positive evidence of disease (such as brain pathology) could be demonstrated.

Probably Meyer was reflecting a growing mood within psychiatry; that mental illness was to be explained and integrated within a growing knowledge of normal behavior, rather than considered simply as another form of physical illness whose symptoms could be taken at face value and tabulated as if for inventory. He undoubtedly was influenced by the exciting new disclosures of psychoanalysis, whose adherents purported to penetrate beneath the surface manifestations of illness to the hidden core of pathology which then could be understood in psychological terms.

To his death, Kraepelin remained a meticulous and objective observer, unwilling to go beyond the mandate of clinical data. Even when psychoanalysis was already luring the attention of the most promising psychiatrists, he wrote: "As I am accustomed to walk on the sure foundations of direct experience, my Philistine conscience of natural science stumbles at every step on objections, considerations and doubts, over which the lightly soaring power of imagination of Freud's disciples carries them without difficulty." (Cited in Braceland, 1957.)

Kraepelin remains the paragon of the objective scientist who refuses to allow his intuitive hunches to interfere with his carefully documented observations. This imposition of order on the chaos that preceded him may be considered the true beginning of modem psychiatry.

The Search for Causes

One of the great appeals that psychoanalysis held for psychiatrists was its insistence that mental illness was not simply the outward manifestation of cerebral pathology, but that its symptoms were psychological in origin and had meaning. Psychoanalysis offered a way of divining that meaning. Kraepelin essentially had disregarded the actual content of his patients' presentations of illness, relying instead on the formal structure of their illness. For Freud, what a patient said and did had meaning and, if one knew how to investigate these behaviors or symptoms, they revealed a sense of logic that could be understood. Beyond Freud's theory of human nature, his formulations of the unconscious, the elaboration of ego defenses, the prepotency of childhood traumas, and the general theory of drives and their derivatives, there is a monumental attempt to seek out the causes of illness. Whether or not any modern student of psychopathology adopts the orthodox viewpoint, it cannot be doubted that he will be influenced by the psychoanalytic search for the hidden motives of behavior.

It was because of this need to prove the existence of disguised motivation that the early psychoanalysts dealt with disorders such as hysteria or obsessive compulsive neurosis, which they believed could demonstrate more readily evidence of unconscious conflicts. Depression, which does not manifest dramatic symptoms that can be interpreted as symbolic of deeper problems, was initially ignored. It was only after Freud had investigated hysteria, obsessions, dreams, parapraxes, jokes, childhood sexuality, and paranoia that he turned his attention to depressive states. When he and his followers did interest themselves in depressive states, their formulations were no less imaginative or revolutionary. The influence of these early psychoanalytic investigations on subsequent psychiatric attitudes toward affective disorders cannot be emphasized strongly enough and consequently will be presented here in rather meticulous detail.

Abraham's Early Contributions

In 1911 Karl Abraham published what may be considered the first psychoanalytic investigation of depression. This pioneer paper must be understood retrospectively within the then prevailing psychoanalytic formulations. In 1911 psychoneurosis was interpreted as a result of repression of libido, so that in this early paper Abraham compares depression to anxiety, which also was believed to be the result of repressed drives. Abraham differentiates between these two states: while anxiety arises when repression prevents the attainment of desired gratification that may still be possible, depression arises when the individual has given up the hope of satisfying his libidinal strivings. Furthermore, in depression the striving toward libidinal satisfaction is so deeply repressed that the individual is unable to feel loved or able to love, despairing of ever achieving emotional intimacy.

Thus Abraham applies the basic doctrine of excessive repression of libido to depression and goes on to confirm this formulation by describing six depressed patients that he treated. These case studies remain classics of description in the psychoanalytic literature.

In discussing these patients, Abraham first draws attention to the similarity between depressed and obsessive patients, a relationship that occurs repeatedly in Abraham's works. In both conditions, Abraham finds a profound ambivalence toward others, in which the striving toward love is blocked by strong feelings of hatred which in turn are repressed because the individual cannot acknowledge his extreme hostility. As with the obsessive, the depressive cannot develop adequately because his feelings of hatred and love constantly interfere with each other. The depressive's interpersonal relations illustrate this repressed hatred which is rooted in blocked libido.

Although the ability to love others is blocked in both conditions because of repression of libido, depressives and obsessives differ radically in the way the blocked impulses find substitutive expression. In the obsessive, repetitive rituals replace the original unacceptable sexual desires. For the depressive, Abraham postulates a peculiar process of projection which he appears to have modeled after the explanation of paranoia that Freud had recently formulated. The internal dynamic processes of the depressive are that he basically feels, "I cannot love people; I have to hate them." This acknowledgement of hatred is unacceptable and must be repressed. Then the hostility is projected onto others and conscious thought is transformed into, "People do not love me; they hate me." This formulation is acceptable and further bolstered by the rationalization that being hated is justified because of some imagined inborn defect.

Abraham goes on to explain other significant aspects of depression on the basis of repression. In a surprisingly modern observation, he states that the massive guilt of the depressive is due to his actual destructive wishes which are kept unconscious. This repressed hostility is clearly manifested in dreams, parapraxes, and other symbolic acts. Abraham asserts that some patients take pride in their sense of guilt, wishing "to be a criminal of the deepest dye, to have more guilt than anyone else put together" (1911, p.

146). He also notes that some depressives appear to enjoy their self-reproaches and to take pleasure in suffering because it allows them to center all of their thoughts on themselves. This self-involvement accounts for the delusions of impoverishment which are symbolic of the emotional deprivation that results from the withdrawal of libido from one's surroundings.

The remainder of Abraham's early contribution concerns itself with mania and with the suitability of depressed individuals for psychoanalytic therapy. Mania is considered to be the overt manifestation of what was repressed during the depressed phase. The blatant expression of love and hate, aptly termed "a frenzy of freedom," which is seen in the manic phase is interpreted as a return to the phase of childhood before the repression of emotion took place. He observes that interviewing a manic adult is much like talking to a five-year old. Abraham admits that he is at a loss to explain why this lifting of repression should occur in some cases and not in others.

The significance of this pioneering work lies in its attempt to bring the affective disorders within the realm of psychoanalytic understanding. In so doing, Abraham limits himself to the formulations available at that time, such as repression and projection. Yet even in this early paper Abraham identifies significant aspects of depressive illness that were missed by previous investigators. He perceives the depressive's ambivalence and his inability to truly love others. He also touches on the depressive's excessive self-concern and his utilization of guilt to draw attention to himself. Finally, Abraham notes the basic hostility which blocks proper emotional growth. In retrospect, what may be lacking here is an appreciation of the role others play in the etiology and maintenance of a depressive episode. The significance of object loss, which later is to become the cardinal event in depression, is not mentioned. Rather, Abraham speculates that affective disorders develop as a result of feelings of being incapable to face the responsibilities of an adult role in society. Ironically, these conclusions were later reached by Adler and others who repudiated much of Freudian theory.

Five years later Abraham published his second contribution to affective disorders, a paper entitled "The First Pregenital Stage of the Libido." The very title of this work indicates the shift that had taken place since the appearance of the preceding paper. In the opening sentences Abraham expresses his intention to give clinical support to the theories Freud had expounded in the third edition of his *Three Essays on the Theory of Sexuality*, which appeared in 1915. Thus Abraham undertakes the task of demonstrating how depression can be integrated into the formulation of regression to a particular libidinal stage of development.

Abraham believes that depression can be understood as a regression to the first psychosexual or oral phase. The similarity between the oral phase and depression is to be found in the mode of libidinal discharge as well as in a characteristic form of object relations. Freud indicated that the orally fixated individual's dominant mode of unconscious relationships was characterized by introjection. Abraham believes that the depressive goes beyond incorporating the psychic object: "In the depths of his unconscious there is a tendency to devour and demolish the object." (1916, p. 276.) It is this unconscious desire to destroy the object orally that accounts for two of the major symptoms of depression: the refusal to take food (that is, equating food with the love object that the individual fears he will destroy) and the fear of starvation (again resulting from a fear of realizing the oral-destructive wishes). Abraham also argues for a seeming antithetical situation; that in some depressives taking food relieves the feeling of depression. However, even in this instance Abraham notes the relationship between depression and orality.

In this contribution the reader begins to detect a drifting away from empirical observation and a subtle yet persistent tendency to force clinical data to fit pre-existing theory. Furthermore, the theory itself becomes more distant from actual observation and thus more difficult to validate empirically. The formulation that depression is an unconscious regression to the first pregenital stage of libido, entailing cannibalistic fantasies as well as defenses against the wishes, is a highly complex formulation that reflects the growing speculative and convoluted nature of psychoanalytic theory. This paper is noteworthy, however, in postulating the role of introjection in depression, which anticipates Freud's later contribution to this subject. Perhaps of greater heuristic value is Abraham's broadening of the libidinal stages to include modes of object relations rather than simply modes of libidinal gratification. In this sense, the pregenital stages become more psychological and less biological, eventually culminating in the work of Sullivan, Fairbairn, and the ego psychologists.

In his third contribution on depression, which appeared in 1924, Abraham continued to trace the origins of the disorder to fixation at the oral stage, although Freud by this time had published his own views on melancholia. Although he again tries to find confirmation for Freud's theories, in this particular publication Abraham seems primarily intent on organizing a typology of illness based on fixations at particular libidinal stages. As before, Abraham begins with the similarity between obsessives and melancholics. Both form ambivalent relationships and show aberrant character traits, such as excessive orderliness and overconcern about money. Abraham speculates that the depressive is actually obsessional during his healthy intervals. He then proposes that both types regress to early pregenital stages; but while the obsessive appears to be satisfied with an unconscious control of the love object, the depressive actually destroys the internalized psychic object. In order to account for this difference, Abraham postulates two subphases of the anal stage: a later phase characterized by withholding, and an earlier phase characterized by expulsion. Abraham suggests that in later life the individual treats his internalized love object the way he originally treated his "earliest piece of private property," namely his feces. He stipulates that the obsessive regresses to the later anal stage, thus maintaining the object; and the depressive regresses to the earlier anal phase, unconsciously expelling and losing the love object. He believes that the obsessive is able to mobilize defenses against further regression that the depressive cannot muster. As a result, the depressive's loss of the internalized love object leaves him with a sense of inner emptiness that he desperately tries to rectify by oral incorporation. Abraham renews his emphasis on oral symptoms in depression: this time he interprets them as efforts to reincorporate the destroyed love object. As proof of his hypothesis, Abraham cites the frequency of coprophilic fantasies in depression, which he interprets not as attempts at self-debasement, but as an unconscious wish to incorporate the anally expelled object by oral means.

Although much of Abraham's effort in this

contribution appears to define further the fixation points for later psychopathology, he also strives to integrate the latest of Freud's theories; in this case the essay *Mourning and Melancholia,* which will be discussed in detail. For the present, it is sufficient to note briefly that Abraham does associate a reparative incorporation of the love object, which is subsequent to loss in depression, with a later ambivalent relationship to this introjected object. This aspect of Freud's theory clearly coincides with Abraham's own contributions. He further agrees that the lost object is treated as part of the ego, so that there is an ambivalent regard toward one's own self, as

exemplified by the contrasting self recriminations during depression and the depressive's feeling superiority during healthy intervals.

Thus having interwoven his own research with current Freudian thinking, Abraham moves on to etiological considerations, in which on clinical grounds his observations again are outstanding. He notes the frequent correlation between the onset of depression and a disappointment in love. Analysis of these cases "invariably" shows that the rejection had a great pathogenic effect because it was sensed in the unconscious to be a repetition of childhood loss of a love object. This early traumatic experience is a potent etiological predisposer to later depressions following any loss. In line with this theory of libidinal development, Abraham states that the childhood disappointment must occur prior to the Oedipal stage when the child's libido is still "narcissistic." That is, object love is tinged with bringing the mental representation of the love object into one's unconscious and treating it as part of one's own self, as well as wishing to destroy it (as described previously). Significant for later theory is Abraham's conclusion, as a result of these theoretical speculations, that since the trauma occurred so early in life it must have been the result of inadequate mothering rather than Oedipal rivalry.

In the last part of this paper, Abraham gives a summary of all three of his contributions on depression and considers various predisposing factors, which are: (1) A constitutional factor in regard to an overaccentuation of oral-eroticism. (2) A special fixation of the libido at the oral level, manifested by disproportionate grievance at frustration and an over-utilization of oral activities (sucking, eating, etc.) in everyday life. (3) A severe injury to infantile narcissism brought about by successive disappointments in love, leading to the childhood prototype of depression called "primal parathymia." (4) The occurrence of the first important disappointment in love before the Oedipal wishes have been overcome. (5) The repetition of the primary disappointment in later life. Throughout, Abraham stresses the importance of ambivalence, be it toward others or toward the incorporated object.

Abraham's final position on depression may be summarized by the following quotation: "When melancholic persons suffer an unbearable disappointment from their love-object they tend to expel that object as though it were feces and to destroy it. They thereupon accomplish the act of introjecting and devouring it—an act which is a specifically melancholic form of narcissistic identification. Their sadistic thirst for vengeance now finds its satisfaction in tormenting the ego —an activity which is in part pleasurable." (1924, p. 469)

In conclusion, Abraham may well be remembered as the person who initiated the psychoanalytic study of depression. He wrote at a time when psychoanalytic theory was fairly uncomplicated, when all psychological illness could be conceived as regression to particular libidinal fixation points.[2] However, in addition to carefully delineating and defining the specific fixations in depression, he stressed the important role of ambivalence, the theory of childhood disappointment in love relationships, and the notion that depression is an adult recapitulation of a childhood trauma. Therefore, even while formulating a somewhat mechanistic metapsychology of melancholia, his clinical acumen allowed him to perceive the powerful interpersonal and psychological aspects of depression.

Mourning And Melancholia

It may be no understatement that Freud's short essay, *Mourning and Melancholia* (1917), changed the course of psychoanalysis. This work stands out because it is the first time that Freud postulates any pathological mechanisms in which the thwarting of sexuality does not play a role. Furthermore, in this paper Freud talks about "object relations" rather than repression, sketches out an agency that later was to become the superego, and also enlarges the role of the ego in pathology. The whole British school of psychoanalysis appears to have its roots in this seminal work in which Freud alters the content of the unconscious to include objects (i.e., mental representations of others) as well as affects and ideas. With this paper, the "mature" works of Freud begin. There is now an appreciation of guilt and aggression as primary motivations, at the expense of blocked erotic expression.

According to Jones (1955), Freud expressed an interest in depression as early as 1914, possibly stimulated by the work of Abraham and Tausk. He wrote *Mourning and Melancholia* in 1915, but it did not appear until 1917 because of the war. The paper is barely twenty pages in length, yet its effect was remarkable; it continues to influence views on depression half a century later, and to reorient much of the course of psychoanalytic investigation. The paper demonstrates flashes of Freud's genius—his ability to see clinical manifestation from a startling new perspective and his power of insightful logical argument.

Freud begins this essay by expressing concern over writing about melancholia, since ultimately this diagnosis may characterize a group of disorders. He further warns the reader that he is basing his findings on a small group of patients who may not warrant generalization.

Freud then compares melancholia with the phenomenon of mourning, noting numerous similarities as well as some critical differences: both share a sense of painful dejection over a loss, a lack of interest in the outside world, the loss of the capacity to love, and an inhibition in activity. However, only melancholia exhibits lowering of self-regard to the extent that there are utterances of self-reproach and an irrational expectation of punishment. Additionally, the melancholic is vague about the nature of his loss, and he is not aware of what has given rise to his dejection. Even when aware of whom he has lost, he is not clear "what it is he has lost in them." This finding leads Freud to believe the loss is internal and unconscious. The loss of self-esteem also points to an internal impoverishment. "In grief," states Freud, "the world has become poor and empty; in melancholia it is the ego itself." How then does Freud account for this inner sense of loss in depression?

He picks up his cue from the inappropriate self-reproaches which (1) are usually moral in content, (2) are grossly unjustified, and (3) are publicly and shamelessly declared. According to Freud this is due to a split in the melancholic's ego, in which one part sets itself over and against the other, judges it critically, and looks upon it as an external object.[3] From these clinical data, Freud speculates that the self-reproaches are not really directed at the self at all, but at some person whom the patient loves, has loved, or ought to have loved. The key to the clinical picture is that the self-reproaches are actually reproaches against a loved object that have been shifted onto the patient's own ego. Therefore the melancholic need have no shame over these reproaches, since they are intended for someone else. Freud shrewdly adds that the melancholic does not really act like a worthless person, despite his protestations, but constantly takes offense as if he had been treated with great injustice. How does this intrapsychic process of shifting an object onto the ego develop?

Freud postulates that in childhood the future melancholic formed an intense object relationship which was undermined because of a disappointment with the loved person. A withdrawal of libidinal investment followed the rupture of the relationship, but the freed libido was not transferred to another object, possibly because of a basically narcissistic type of relating. Instead this libido was withdrawn into the ego. However, an identification was made between part of the ego and the forsaken object, and this ego identification absorbs the libido. Freud describes this process with his famous and dramatic words: "Thus the shadow of the object fell upon the ego, so that the latter could henceforth be criticized by a special mental faculty like an object, like the forsaken object." Therefore the internalized effigy of the lost object becomes subject to the ambivalent feelings of the individual and is subject to the scorn and hatred that would have been directed at the lost object. This, then, is the intrapsychic predisposition to melancholia.

Later losses reactivate the primal loss and cause the patient's fury to be vented at the original disappointing object, which has been fused with part of the patient's own ego. In extreme cases, the sadism is so virulent that the individual wishes to destroy the internal effigy of the object totally and commits suicide. For most melancholics, sufficient gratification is obtained by vilifying the effigy, which clinically appears as self-reproachment. When this fury has been spent or the object effigy abandoned as being no longer of value, the illnesses passes until another loss reinitiates the entire process. In some patients there is a sudden release of libido from the internal effigy and this surplus of energy is expended in manic behavior. In mania, the ego has mastered this internalized rage and thrust the problem aside; in melancholia, the ego is beaten by the critical agency and continues to be subjected to its anger.

In conclusion, Freud stipulates three conditioning factors in melancholia: the loss of the object, a high degree of ambivalence, and a regression of libido into the ego. While all three are necessary, only the last is specific to melancholia.

In retrospect, Freud's short essay is a masterpiece of clinical investigation and logical deduction. Yet it may have raised more difficulties than it resolved. The essay proposed an entirely new model of illness: the expression of affect toward an incorporated object (although Abraham, in his investigation of depression along the lines of libidinal regression, gave a similar description).[4] This formulation has become increasingly difficult to prove or corroborate by clinical evidence. Therapists for decades have induced their depressed patients, with little success, to express anger so as to deflect it from the internalized effigy. Some depressives have not evidenced the crucial selfreproaches. Depressed individuals do not uniformly present a history of past or current loss. Therefore Freud's bold and imaginative formulation does not appear to have survived the test of time.

The formulation has also had its problems from a theoretical standpoint. The critical agency has become the superego which vents its anger at the ego in all neurotic disorders, not just in melancholia. The concept of the introjection of the disappointing object has gained wider application, especially in the work of the Kleinians, so that it also is no longer specific for melancholia. Later orthodox formulations on depression, which will be discussed below, have essentially discarded the introject hypothesis in favor of one viewing depression as a result of a felt disparity between the ego ideal and the actual self.

Nevertheless *Mourning and Melancholia* remains a classic in psychoanalytic literature. Freud was able to see that in depression one person has deeply affected the mental state of another, and that the loss of this person results in an *internal* loss for the depressive. He thus recognized the interpersonal nature of the disorder and the close relationship between maintenance of self-esteem and maintenance of a successful relationship. He also attempted to show that depressives are predisposed to their disorder by childhood events, usually prior disappointments with significant others which lead to a pervasive ambivalence in all their relationships. Finally, in his insightful way he managed to see through the specious selfreproaches of some depressives, noting that in the end they also punish the external, loved other by becoming ill.

Further Traditional Developments

Freud did not devote another complete work to depression, but he did allude to it in a number of his later writings. In his book *Group Psychology and the Analysis of Ego* (1921), in which Freud discusses the forces that account for the cohesion of a group, he also briefly recapitulates his formulation on melancholia. Freud examines the relationships of the ego to the ego ideal, as well as to idealized others. Here he describes mania as a fusion of the ego and the ego ideal so that the former is free of criticism from the latter. In melancholia the ego, having identified with the disappointing object, is subject to the ego ideal's attacks. It becomes clear that the ego ideal soon will be recast as the superego.

Finally in *The Ego and the Id* (1922), which outlines the major revision of the structural theory, Freud returns to the mechanism of introjection or identification with a cathected object. He states that introjection is a much more general process than he had previously considered it to be. The mechanism of incorporating a frustrating object may in fact be the manner by which the child's ego gradually develops its specific character, as a "precipitate" of abandoned, internalized objects. Therefore, identification or incorporation becomes the major mechanism for dealing with objects that are lost, abandoned, or frustrating. This internalization becomes the manner through which a loss is undone in the unconscious.

Having shown that an ego ideal (or superego) is ubiquitous, as is the process of internalizing abandoned objects, Freud now proposes that melancholia results from an extreme discord between the superego and the ego, with the superego venting its rage against a seemingly helpless ego. As for why the melancholic should have such a harsh and powerful superego, Freud relies on his newly formulated hypothesis of the death instinct and also notes that if aggression is not expressed outwardly, it will be turned against the self.

Freud's final revision of his theory of melancholia in *The Ego and the Id* is of crucial importance, for it essentially negates much of what had been written earlier in *Mourning and Melancholia*. Yet Freud's later statement is often ignored and the earlier work later taken as his last word on depression. Freud dramatically restates this later view of melancholia in his *New Introduction Lectures* (1933): "No sooner have we got used to the idea of the superego . . . then we are faced with a clinical picture which throws into strong relief the severity, and even cruelty, of this function, and the vicissitudes through which its relations with the ego may pass. I refer to the condition of melancholia" (1933, p. 87).

The revision of psychoanalytic theory that was brought about by the effect of the structural theory on psychodynamics was most thoroughly and creatively described by Sandar Rado. In a highly influential paper (1928), Rado considered depression and mania in terms of the interlocking relationships between the ego, the superego, and the love object. Rado observed that prior to the onset of an episode of depression, the individual goes through a period of arrogant and embittered rebellion. Rado explained that this phase of affective disorder is easily overlooked in that it passes quickly and is soon overshadowed by more blatant melancholic symptomatology. This phase is typical—although an exaggeration—of the depressive manner of treating the love object during healthy intervals. As soon as the depressive is sure of the other's love, he treats his beloved with a "sublime nonchalance," gradually progressing to a domineering and tyrannical control of the love object. This behavior may ultimately push away the loved other, who will not tolerate this mistreatment any longer. When and if this loss occurs, the individual lapses into depression.

The reason for this response to object loss resides in the peculiar personality structure of the depression-prone individual. Although he bullies and tests the love object, the depressive desperately needs the other's constant nurturance. He needs to be showered with love and admiration and will not tolerate frustration of this need. This type of individual appears inordinately reliant on others for narcissistic gratification and for maintaining self-esteem. Even trivial disappointments appear to cause an upset in the depressive's self-regard and to result in his immediate effort to relieve subsequent discomfort. To quote Rado, "They have a sense of security and comfort only when they feel themselves loved, esteemed, and encouraged. Even when they display an approximately normal activity in the gratification of their instincts and succeed in realizing their aims and ideals, the self-esteem largely depends on whether they do or do not meet with approbation and recognition" (1928). As a result of this need, the depressive become exquisitely skillful in extracting demonstration of love from others. However, as just described, he will push the test of love to the limits of tolerance in any relationship during periods of security and relative health. During periods of depression which occur after the object have been driven away, the individual resorts to a different method of coercion. He becomes remorseful and contrite, begging for forgiveness, and hopes to regain the lost object through inducing pity and guilt.

This pattern of hostility-guilt-contrition is explained by Rado as arising in early childhood when the child learned that he could win forgiveness and regain the all-meaningful love of the mother by appropriate remorseful behavior. This guilt-atonement sequence is traced by Rado to an earlier progression of rage-hungerdrinking at the mother's breast. Rado strongly emphasizes that the desire to be nursed at the mother's breast is at the core of melancholia and its unconscious persistence into adult life accounts for both the oral fixation described by Abraham and the need for external emotional nurturance. Ultimately the depressives desires to be passive are satisfied by an all-giving other whom he can control and tyrannize.

If the depressive cannot win back the love of the lost object, he progresses to a more malignant form of melancholia in which the interpersonal drama is replaced by an intrapsychic struggle. Here Rado shows the influence of the structural theory by postulating that in severe (possibly psychotic) depression, external objects are given up and the ego seeks forgiveness from the superego which has replaced the love object. Therefore the selfreproaches of the severe melancholic are understandable in terms of the ego's hoping to attain the love of the superego by appropriate repentive behavior.

Rado believes that this intrapsychic stage of depression is an extension of the basic psychodynamics but at a different level; he assumes that both ego and superego were originally formed by incorporation of aspects of a love object, and the ego now seeks love and forgiveness from an internalized rather than external love object. He postulates that in childhood, when self-esteem was primarily derived from positive parental responses, the child gradually internalized this esteem-giving parent into an intrapsychic agency—namely, the superego. However, Rado speculates that there was actually a double introjection. Due to the immature cognitive abilities of the child, the parent was experienced as totally good (when giving pleasure) or totally bad (when frustrating needs), and not as a complete person who could be good and bad at the same time. Rado believes that the good object, whose love was strongly desired, was incorporated into the superego, while the bad, frustrating object was internalized into the ego which became the "whipping boy" of the good object. The depressive continues to desire the love of the good internalized object, and the outward manifestations of the ego's attempt to gain the love through contrition and atonement make up the clinical manifestations of melancholia. Through self-denial and selfpunishment, the ego eventually regains the love of the superego and the episode of depression resolves itself with a resulting rise in the selfesteem and a renewed interest in external objects.

The significant aspects of Rado's theory are that depression represents a process of repair and a period of atonement for having driven away the needed object. At first there is an attempt to coerce an external object into granting forgiveness and love. If this interpersonal maneuver fails, the disorder progresses to an intrapsychic level where the struggle takes place between the ego and superego. The influence of Abraham's notion of controlling and losing the object is evident, as well as Freud's ideas of a harsh superego and anger turned toward an object that has been introjected into the ego. Rado transforms these previous formulations to fit the concepts of the structural theory, but he also adds much original thought, such as the depressive's need of others to bolster his self-esteem and the repetition of a childhood pattern of rage-atonement. Rado further tries to place degrees of severity of depression on a continuum with the same basic causative mechanisms. He brings his formulation closer to clinical data by demonstrating how the melancholic episode eventually clears by itself by gaining atonement from the superego or by reinstating a relationship with the love object. The weaknesses of Rado's theory appear to be his basic speculation of a double introjection in childhood, and his treatment of the intrapsychic structural agencies in a rather anthropomorphic manner.

Almost a quarter of a century later, Rado (1951) returned to the study of depression after he had reformulated psychoanalysis from the standpoint of psychobiological adaptation to the environment. In this later personal view, he conceived of psychopathology as the inappropriate persistence of infantile adaptive patterns into adult life. With particular reference to depression, Rado still maintained that the depressive manifestations are attempts to restore a sense of being cared for which is analogous to the security that the infant feels at its mother's breast. The symptoms of the adult melancholic were interpreted as patterned after the infant's "loud cry for help." For example, the depressive's fear of impoverishment, and his hypochondriasis and gastro-intestinal complaints, were equated with the infant's fear of not getting sufficient nutrients. In addition, Rado still interpreted the whole purpose of depression as an unconscious expiation which aims at restoring the lost love object. At this point Rado recapitulated his earlier exposition of pushing the love object to the limits of tolerance and then punishing oneself for the loss. However, Rado added some new dimensions to his 1928 theory. He now believed that the depressive may despise himself because of his own weakness and because he cannot get his own way through anger. The dilemma of the melancholic is to be torn between coercive rage and submissive fear. In a manner reminiscent of Abraham's emphasis on ambivalence, Rado declared that the depressive wishes to express tremendous anger at the love object, but he is prevented from overt manifestations of hostility because of his dependency on the love object. When this balance is upset and the depressive loses the object, he is said to vent his rage on himself and simultaneously revert to the old pattern of atonement in the hopes of winning back the love object.

Rado calls this reaction to loss "a process of miscarried repair." For the healthy person, the experience of loss is a challenge which marshals his resources to continue life without the needed object or to take appropriate steps to rectify the loss. In the depressive individual, a loss "presses the obsolete adaptive pattern of alimentary maternal dependence into service and by this regressive move, it incapacitates the patient still more." Therefore depression from the standpoint of adaptational psychodynamics is a persistent but no longer effective mode of reaction to the loss of love.

Finally, Rado adds that he is less impressed with the role of actual environmental loss. At times the loss may be insignificant, but it is exaggerated by the patient. At other times the loss may be totally unconscious and outside the awareness of the individual. And, like Sullivan, he believes that in some cases no loss occurs but the patient invents a precipitating event to rationalize becoming depressed. Rado concludes that depression can be brought on by whatever succeeds in arousing guilty fear and regressive dependency—i.e., the maladaptive repair sequence. Melancholia is significant as a pathological reparative process and not for what may elicit it. By 1951 Rado's interests had clearly shifted from classical psychodynamics to describing both healthy and pathological responses to stress in which adaptive, appropriate, and mature patterns were the

criteria of health, and maladaptive, anachronistic, and childhood patterns were the criteria of pathology.

Depression and Ego Psychology

When Fenichel's encyclopedic summary of psychoanalysis appeared in 1945, he devoted a chapter to depression in which he discussed the current psychoanalytic views on the disorder. In this work Fenichel drew upon the works of others in enumerating the various factors in depression. He mentioned the "pathognomic introject" formulation initiated by Freud, the oral fixation as postulated by Abraham, and the incessant need for love as described by Rado. In this last regard, Fenichel referred to depressives as love addicts who insist on a constant flow of benevolence and care little for the actual personality or needs of the bestower of this love. Fenichel also agreed with Rado's differentiation of neurotic depression as a state where love from an external object is sought, from psychotic depression as a state where external objects have been renounced and love is demanded from an internal agency. However, he believed this difference to be less absolute in that neurotic depressives try to appease the superego, and severe melancholics have not totally withdrawn from the object world but hope that an all-giving other will fulfill their craving for love. In reviewing all of these theories in detail, Fenichel strongly emphasized another aspect of depression which was to greatly influence the course of later psychoanalytic thinking.

This aspect that Fenichel conceived to be central to the whole problem of depression was the fall in self-esteem. Previous authors had alluded to a lowering of self-regard as present in depression, but Fenichel appeared to make the fall in self-esteem the key factor. Fenichel wrote: "A person who is fixated on the state where his self-esteem is regulated by external supplies or a person whose guilt feelings motivate him to regress to this state vitally needs these supplies. He goes through this world in a condition of perpetual greediness. If his narcissistic needs are not satisfied, his self-esteem diminishes to a danger point" (1945, p. 387).

The centrality of the regulation of selfesteem and its relationship to depression has redirected the line of psychoanalytic investigation into affective disorders. The subsequent importance of the ego can be appreciated when it is understood that it is the ego that allegedly gauges self-esteem by measuring the discrepancy between the actual state of self and a desired ego ideal. Self-esteem is believed to be the felt expression of this disparity.

This approach to depression has been taken by three theorists: Jacobson, Bibring, and Sandler. Their views continue to influence current thinking on depression strongly. Although proposing quite different overall systems of thought, each selected self-esteem regulation as central to depression and also roughly equated self-esteem as the felt discrepancy between the actual self and a desired ideal state.

The first of these theorists to be considered is Edith Jacobson, who has written extensively on depression and whose interest in severely disturbed manic-depressive patients extends over half a century. Her writings are very complex and her explanation of depression is embedded in her own theory of psychological development. Briefly, Jacobson (1954) postulates that the mind develops out of an undifferentiated matrix by the gradual formation on self and object representations, roughly meaning the internalized image of oneself and other individuals. Each of these representations can be cathected by libido, aggressive, or neutralized energy. These "cathectic shifts" account for one's feeling about oneself and others, depending on which representation is the recipient of each type of energy. In infancy a devaluation of others (an aggressive cathexis of the object representation) due to frustration is said to result also in a devaluation of the self, since the self still is fused with the representation of others. In an early paper (1946) Jacobson describes the effect of early disappointments on the belief in parental omnipotence, and the subsequent devaluation of parental images. This disappointment leads to a concurrent devaluation of the self and a primary childhood depression which is reactivated by adult disillusionments. Similarly, the infant's alleged grandiosity is said to be a result of selfrepresentation being fused with an idealized (libidinally cathected) object representation.

Other more traditional constructs utilized by Jacobson are the ego ideal and the superego. The former is defined as the residual of narcissistic strivings in the child which the ego constantly seeks to measure up to in terms of standards. The latter is defined as a system that regulates the libidinous and aggressive cathexis to the self-representations, independent of the outside world. In healthy individuals the superego develops into an abstract, depersonified agency, but in pathology the superego is not well formed, still being tied to persons from the past and apt to be confused with objects in the outside world. This lack of differentiation of the superego interferes with appropriate cathexis of the self-representation and also affects self-esteem.

In depression there is an aggressive cathexis of the self, with a poor differentiation of the superego and a lack of adequate separation of object representations from the childhood parental ideal. In this sense depression can be seen economically as a problem of cathectic investment, and structurally as a lack of differentiation. For Jacobson the basic conflict in all affective disorders is as follows: When frustration is encountered, rage is aroused and leads to hostile attempts to gain the desired gratification. However, if the ego is unable (for external or internal reasons) to achieve this goal, aggression is turned to the self-image (1971, p. 183). This deflation of the self-image causes a greater disparity between it and the ideal selfimage, leading to a feeling of low self-esteem. The depressed individual then may defensively try to fuse with an omnipotent object (mania) or turn to a new object to replenish libidinal supplies in order to raise self-esteem.

In describing a severely depressed patient, Jacobson states: "His self-representations retained the infantile conception of a helpless self drawing its strength from a powerful, ideal love object. He tried to keep the image of this love object hypercathected, by constantly depriving the self-image of its libidinal cathexis and pouring it on the object image. He then had to bolster his self-image again by a reflux of libido from the image of his love object" (1971, p. 235). In this passage, Jacobson is describing how the patient needed to relate to an overvalued other to maintain self-esteem. The text is quoted to give the reader a sense of her insistence on utilizing drive theory in describing clinical pathology. Jacobson has, in fact, criticized other theorists for their neglect of the economic aspects of psychoanalytic theory in their formulations.

She continues to rely on drive dynamics in describing the further course of depression. According to Jacobson, if the depressive fails to find a new love object that can replenish libidinal supplies to his self-image, he then will turn to a powerful but sadistic love object in the hope of gaining strength, if not love. If this last-ditch effort also fails, she postulates that the individual will retreat from relationships with the outside world and will reanimate an internal primitive and powerful image from the past. This powerful, internal object-representation merges with the superego, which becomes personified, and the true object representations, which have become deflated, merge with the selfrepresentation. In this manner the last step in the depressive progression is the familiar retreat from the world of objects and the reconstitution of the love object in the superego. Thus while Jacobson follows the traditional view of psychotic depression as characterized (in contrast to neurotic depression) by a shifting from external relationships to strictly intrapsychic cathexes, she also believes that an as yet undiscovered neurological defect is necessary for the development of psychotic depression.

These few words cannot do justice to the complexity of Jacobson's views on the regulation of moods and self-esteem. Her system is an attempt at a "purification" of psychoanalytic constructs which she has elaborately defined and differentiated. However, in describing her clinical work, doubts arise as to her own ability to adhere to her strict definitions and many of the concepts become anthropomorphized. Significant about her formulations may be her attempt to assimilate ego psychology and drive theory together with her own brand of an objects-relations approach. It may well be that this synthesis is not possible in every detail when applied to actual clinical experience as opposed to purely theoretical speculation.

Nevertheless Jacobson presents a comprehensive analysis of depression built on cathectic shifts of aggressive energy and libido between self and object representations, as well as on the fusion of intrapsychic structures—all the while considering the regulation of selfesteem to be the major problem of depression. In summary, Jacobson should be read as both a clinician and a metapsychologist. In her clinical work her insights are remarkable, and her work on the therapy of depression is outstanding. As for her metapsychology, it remains a theoretical attempt to reduce clinical data to speculative hypothetical constructs. It is almost as if she were describing two theories, the clinical and the hypothetical, and the reader is free to follow her formulations as far as they coincide with his own convictions.

In contrast to Jacobson's complicated metapsychology, Bibring's (1953) theory is a paradigm of simplicity and clarity. He presents brief vignettes of patients who were depressed following a variety of life events. Despite differences in circumstances and secondary symptomatology, all of these individuals presented a basic common pattern. All felt helpless in the face of superior powers or were unavoidably confronted with the sense of being a failure, and all had suffered a blow to selfesteem. Bibring concludes: "From this point of view, depression can be defined as the emotional expression (indication) of a state of helplessness and powerlessness of the ego, irrespective of what may have caused the breakdown of the mechanisms which established his self-esteem" (1953, p. 24). Further central features of depression, according to Bibring, are the ego's acute awareness of its actual or imaginary helplessness and its strong narcissistic aspirations which it cannot fulfill.

While these two factors—the sense of helplessness and the discrepancy between one's actual situation and a wished for set of ideal circumstances —have been mentioned by others, Bibring's originality is that he views this combination of events as resulting in a tension within the ego itself and not in an intersystemic conflict (for example, between ego and superego) or in a conflict between the ego and the environment. For Bibring, depression is the emotional correlate of a particular state of the ego. By considering depression in this light, Bibring compares it with anxiety and concludes that both are primary experiences which cannot be broken down any further. Although it seems a somewhat simple observation, this view of depression has far-reaching consequences: it unites normal, neurotic, and psychotic depressions as being due to the same basic mechanism. Furthermore, by viewing depression as a primary ego state that is possible in everyone, this formulation shifts the importance from the internal structure of depression to the environmental and characterological factors that facilitate the depressive response. Therefore Bibring mentions that some individuals are predisposed to depression because of unrealistic aspirations which cannot be fulfilled or because of excessive past experiences of feeling, and perhaps being, helpless. Finally, if depression is a simple, basic experiential state like anxiety, it is to be expected that individuals may form certain defenses against it or even that it may serve a useful purpose (again, like anxiety) when experienced in mild forms. Therefore the symptoms of depression itself are not reparative (as postulated by Rado and others), but other symptoms developed in reaction to depression may well be so.

Sandler and Joffe (1965) have reached conclusions similar to Bibring's as a result of clinical work with disturbed children, and from theoretical investigations of the meaning of some psychoanalytic concepts such as the superego and the ego ideal. They also view depression to be a basic affect (like anxiety) that is experienced when an individual believes he has lost something that was essential to his state of wellbeing and he feels unable to undo this loss. Sandler and Joffe further postulate that what is lost in depression is a feeling of narcissistic integrity, and not any specific "object." They state, "When a love-object is lost, what is really lost, we believe, is the state of well-being implicit, both psychologically and biologically, in the relationship with the object" (1965, p. 91). While acknowledging their debt to Bibring, Sandler and Joffe believe that "loss of selfesteem" is too elaborate and intellectual a concept to indicate the primal nature of this reaction which, for example, can be seen in children. Rather, they conceive of depression as the feeling of having been deprived of an ideal state, the vehicle of which was often but not exclusively a relationship with another person.

Sandler and Joffe also differentiate between depression as a basic psychobiological response that automatically results from the situations described, and clinical depression which is a further elaboration or abnormal persistence of the basic unpleasant reaction. The initial response is analogous to a sort of "mental pain," which reflects a discrepancy between the actual state of the self and an ideal state of psychological wellbeing. If the individual feels helpless, resigned, or impotent in the face of the painful situation, then he experiences the affective response of depression. In regard to the hypothesis of depression as anger turned toward the self, they suggest that the initial loss generates rage; but this hostility is not allowed expression or is directed against a self which is disliked for its lack of effectiveness. Therefore there is blocked aggression in depressed individuals, according to Sandler and Joffe, but this finding does not necessarily conform to the Freudian introject formulation. Finally, like Bibring, Sandler and Joffe perceive that the initial psychobiological depressive reaction elicits defenses and does not uniformly proceed to a clinical depressive episode. It may also have a salutary effect in the manner that Freud proposed for signal anxiety.

Ego psychology has altered the traditional psychoanalytic thinking on depression, stressing that the ego's awareness of painful discrepancies is central to depression and its cardinal feature is a fall in self-esteem. Jacobson has incorporated this view into a complex system that relies heavily on metaphysical constructs and drive theory. Bibring, Sandler, and Joffe, on the other hand, have utilized the insights of ego psychology to simplify the traditional view of depression and reduce it to a basic psychobiological experiential state that cannot be explained by or further reduced to intersystemic conflicts.

While this shift in orientation appears to be closely aligned to clinical data, questions arise as to its adequacy in explaining or describing a depressive episode. Numerous authors outside the orthodox camp, such as Sullivan or Homey, for decades have postulated a fall in self-esteem to be basic to almost all psychopathology, so that the ego psychologists have actually just come around to a previously well-documented position. If this view is correct, then poor selfesteem regulation is a necessary but not sufficient explanation for depression since it occurs in other disorders. Rather, what appears necessary is an explanation of how depression differs from other syndromes that are also a reaction to low self-esteem. Jacobson has attempted such an explanation with her utilization of the concept of an aggressive cathexis of the self-representation. However, as stated earlier, her system requires accepting an elaborate metapsychology which does not always appear to fit clinical observations. Nevertheless, the "self-esteem regulation" approach to depression does allow for this disorder to be compared to other states of pathology that result from a fall in self-esteem and for the utilization of specific mechanisms that produce depression in certain individuals to be investigated.

The Contributions of Melanie Klein

Although Melanie Klein considered her contributions to be a logical extension of orthodox psychoanalysis, it has become clear over the years that she was an innovative thinker who originated a unique system of psychodynamic interpretation that ultimately crystallized into a separate group of disciples loosely called the British school of psychoanalysis. Her major concerns, which grew out of her first-hand clinical experience with severely disturbed children and her personal exposure to the thinking of Karl Abraham, were the earliest stages of psychic life and the predominant role of ambivalence in psychopathology. Her contributions to depression can be understood only in the context of her general system, so a cursory sketch of it is presented here.[5]

Klein postulates two basic developmental stages in the first year of life which she calls "positions." The first is the schizo-paranoid position, and it is characterized by a particular perception of part-objects rather than of realistic whole objects. For example, the infant during this stage of development is said to conceive of the breast as separate from the mother. In addition, the "good" feeding breast is perceived to be a different object than the "bad" nongiving breast. In this manner, the child resolves the problem of ambivalence by "splitting" the whole object into separate good and bad part objects that do not belong to the same person. In addition to sensing that these good and bad objects exist in the external world, the infant internalizes the objects (because of poor selfenvironment differentiation) so that they become "internal objects" within the psyche. According to Klein, the infant is frightened that the bad internalized objects will destroy the good internalized objects. He resolves this conflict by projecting the bad objects back into the environment in order to safeguard his inner sense of goodness. In this manner, the child senses danger from without, called "persecutory anxiety," although the child has himself projected the bad inner objects into the environment: hence the term "paranoid position." Initially Klein believed that the danger to the good objects came from the child's own innate aggression which was a deflection of the death instinct, and this struggle to ward off the bad objects was independent of environmental factors. Subsequent theorists have taken a less nativistic view; they believe that the quality of maternal care affects the balance of good and bad objects.

The second position is called the "depressive position." It is said to occur at about four to five months of age, when the infant's cognitive abilities mature sufficiently and he can begin to perceive realistic whole objects. At this stage the child realizes that the good and bad breasts both belong to the same mother, and he has to deal with the conflict of external figures being the sources of both pain and pleasure.

Similarly he must deal with his own ambivalence and can no longer project his hostility onto the environment. The crisis at this stage is the child's fear that his aggression, which he now recognizes as his own, will destroy the good objects both external and internal. Thus the major dread is called "depressive" anxiety; it relates to the child's fear that he himself has caused the loss or destruction of his sense of well-being (good objects).

There are a variety of ways in which the child can deal with the depressive position. One is to become inhibited, depressed, and fearful of action lest he destroy the good objects. Another is to deny the value of the good objects and to insist that he needs no other object than himself (the so-called manic defense). Finally, the healthy resolution is for the child to realize that although his actions or wishes may have temporarily caused the loss of the good objects, these can be reinstated by appropriate restitutive maneuvers. In this way the individual acknowledges his responsibilities for his hostile feelings (he does not project them onto others), and at the same time he has the assurance that his hostility is not so massively destructive, that through appropriate behavior he can regain a good feeling about himself (i.e., the inner good objects). Kleinians have gone as far as speculating that most, if not all, adult creative endeavors are symbolic reparative productions for childhood destructive wishes.

This brief summary does not do justice to the complexity of the Kleinian system, but it may allow an appreciation of her conceptualization of depression. For Klein, depression holds a central place in psychopathology because it is seen as underlying many other clinical entities. As such, her position is similar to Sandler and to Bibring in viewing depression as an almost basic state which has to be defended against in either an abnormal or healthy fashion. However, in Klein's system depression takes on a new and less specific meaning; it is a normal stage of development, a specific form of anxiety, and the "depressive conflict" can be seen as underlying most neurotic illness (in contrast to the schizoparanoid position, which appears to describe schizophrenic states). Winnicott has, in fact, considered the depressive position as a developmental achievement in that the individual accepts responsibility for his anger and is able to tolerate ambivalence.

Klein (1940) did attempt to relate the symptoms of clinical depression to her system, proposing that in the "internal warfare" of inner objects, depression is experienced when the ego identifies itself with the sufferings of the good objects subjected to the attacks of bad objects and the id. She also relates the suffering of the adult melancholic to the nursing child's feelings of guilt and remorse over experiencing conflict between love and uncontrollable hatred toward its good objects. The most significant predisposition to melancholia, according to Klein, is the failure of the infant to establish its loved, good object with the ego. This accounts for a lifelong feeling of "badness" which is not projected outward, but which is incorporated into the self-image.

Klein's system has been rightly accused of extreme reification; that is, the hypothetical internal objects are talked of as actual concrete entities. There have also been criticisms that she ascribes all sorts of sophisticated abilities to the young infant, that she stresses pathology too much in everyday behavior, and that she fits all the patient's therapeutic productions in her system in a procrustean fashion. Finally, she has been accused of totally ignoring the environment and focusing only on the innate unfolding of instinctual processes and later on the inner battle between internalized objects. As for this last criticism, her followers—especially Fairbairn, Winnicott, and Guntrip—have increasingly taken cognizance of environmental factors so that the term "object relations" refers to external as well as internal objects. Lately Kleinian formulations have surprisingly found favor with family therapists who have expanded them to account for interactions between family members. In this regard, Slipp (1976) has combined family transactional theory with Kleinian psychodynamics in a comprehensive exposition of the development of the melancholic patient. Slipp enumerates various roles that are forced on the child according to the parental introject that the parents project onto the child. These projected parental introjects are often contradictory so that the child grows up in a conflict over his own behavior. For example, the child is pressured to succeed in order to salvage the family's image, yet his successes are sabotaged because the parents fear the child's ultimate independence from them. Slipp further elaborates how the child gradually evolves a depressive character and specific defenses in reaction to these parental interactions. He describes the adult depressive's main struggle as turning the bad parental introject into a good introject so that he can feel worthwhile.

In summary, Klein advanced the study of depression by stressing the fear of action for loss of needed objects, the lack of early incorporation of good objects, and the important role of guilt and hostility rather than libidinal transformation. However, she continued to be locked within the intrapsychic world (as have been most of the other authors considered so far), and to virtually ignore the real impact of interchange with significant others in the predisposition to depression. Attention will now be directed to an appreciation of these interpersonal and cultural factors.

The Interpersonal and Cultural Schools

Since Freud's fateful decision to treat his patients' reminiscences as childhood fantasies rather than as true—albeit distorted— memories, traditional psychoanalysis has taken a specific perspective on human behavior, considering mainly the intrapsychic at the expense of cultural and interpersonal influences. Freud was obviously aware of the importance of human interaction in the regulation of psychic functioning, but he preferred to deal with relationships in terms of object representations within the mind which were subject to instinctual cathexes either in harmony or in battle with other internal structures. He chose to conceptualize both pathological and normal development as the unfolding of innate forces and to give minimal regard to societal or interpersonal influences. An exception was made for experiences in childhood because they fit into his prearranged psychosexual stages which, however, were conceived of as means of obtaining gratification rather than as ways of relating to others. Another obvious exception was the boy's identification with his father at the termination of the Oedipal conflict.

In a similar unilateral perspective, Freud saw adult problems as clear repetitions of childhood events without giving appropriate weight to the individual's current situation, the actual effect of life vicissitudes on adult experience as independent of past history, and— most important—the effect of the patient's behavior, including his illness, on those around him. In reaction to Freud's intrapsychic, biological, and mechanistic metapsychology, opposing points of view became organized into various schools, each stressing a particular objection. Some of these reactions may loosely be called the interpersonal, the cultural, and the existential psychoanalytic schools of thought. While many of these schools rejected orthodox psychoanalysis completely, others attempted a synthesis of Freudian doctrine with other points of view. Finally, even within the orthodox psychoanalytic circles there has been a gradual evolution toward these newer formulations which originally were considered deviant and radical.

The first comprehensive works which dealt extensively with nonintrapsychic factors in the study of depression were the two publications on manic-depressives by Cohen and her coworkers (1949, 1954), undertaken by the Washington School of Psychiatry, and utilizing a predominantly Sullivanian orientation. These studies are noteworthy; they consider the family atmosphere in which the future depressive grows up, the effect of the patient on others, and the overall depressive personality.

In terms of family background, Cohen's group found that in each of their twelve cases the family set itself, or was forced by others to be, apart from the general community. In some cases the separation was due to membership in a minority religion, and in others the separation was on the basis of economic differences or chronic family illness. In every case the family felt its isolation keenly and attempted to gain acceptance from neighbors. Toward this end, the children were expected to conform to a high standard of "good" behavior and to achieve in order to undo the family's alleged lower status. Cohen et al. concluded that using the child as a instrument for improving the family's social position devalues the child as a person in his own right. Even in families who thought themselves better than their neighbors, the child's accomplishments were regarded as serving to enhance the family's reputation rather than to instill a sense of achievement and selfpride in the child.

The mother was found to be the stronger parent, demanding obedience and excellence. The father, on the other hand, was often economically and socially unsuccessful. Within the home he was subjected to the mother's criticism and depreciation. The patients remembered their fathers as weak but lovable, giving them the implicit message, "Do not be like me." The mother was seen as the reliable though less accepting and loving parent. The example of the father was a dramatic reminder to the children of what might happen to them if they failed to achieve the high goals set by the mother. Cohen et al. further investigated the early childhood development of the manic-depressive and found a consistent pattern in which the mother enjoyed her relationship with the child when he was a helpless infant, but resented his individuating and independent behavior as a toddler. The mothers liked the utter dependence of an infant but could not cope with the rebelliousness of a young child, so they managed to control the unruly behavior by threats of abandonment. In contrast to Freud and Abraham, the Washington group did not find a history of a childhood loss or a childhood depressive episode (Abraham's primal parathymia); rather, they found the omnipresent threat of loss if normal, spontaneous behavior was expressed.

The later childhood development of the patients revealed that they often had held a special or favorite position within the family because of either superior endowment or greater efforts to please. This favoritism was based only on the ability to achieve and not on any true concern for the individual as separate from the family unit. As a result of this upbringing, the child grew up as a manipulator, viewing human relationships as a means of promoting his own desired ambitions. At the same time he suffered from extreme envy of others and a fear of competitiveness which manifested itself as a specious underselling of himself in order to disarm others and to obtain their needed support.

These childhood experiences were said to result in a definite adult personality structure uniformly found in the twelve manic-depressives studied. One outstanding feature was the manicdepressive's lack of appreciating another person as separate from his own needs. Other people were seen almost as pieces of property which belonged to him, and from whom he could demand continuing support. As the same time there was a fear of abandonment so that the manic-depressive shunned confrontations or direct competition. Most were diligent, hardworking, compulsive individuals (between attacks), hoping to please others in order to make dependent demands on them. Despite hard work, there was little evidence of creativity; rather, these patients tended to take on the values or opinions of authority figures in the environment.

Cohen did not find striking evidence of hostility although she and her associates describe how the patient's incessant demands and lack of empathy could create a hostile impression on those around him. In general, the Washington group felt that the most constant factor was an inner sense of emptiness and a constant need for support which external figures had to rectify. This latter demand for an external figure to meet inner needs was what predisposed the individual to clinical decompensation if the relationship with the needed other was terminated. The actual depressive episode was interpreted as the external manifestation of an attempt to win back the needed other. If hope of renewing the relationship was lost, the depression progressed to a psychotic state unless a manic denial of the needed other supervened.

The Washington group also described specific problems in the therapy of manicdepressive individuals. One obstacle is the overwhelming dependency on the therapist that eventually develops. The other is the "stereotyped response"; that is, the patient's inability to view the therapist objectively, but only as a stereotyped repetition of a parental figure. The therapist is utilized as:

1. An object to be manipulated for purposes of gaining sympathy and reassurance.

2. A moral authority who can be coerced into giving approval.

3. A critical or rejecting authority who will not give real but only token approval.

This last conceptualization is often quite accurate since these patients readily alienate their therapists with suffocating demands. These distortions of the manic-depressive are interpreted as a fixation at Klein's part-object stage, so that the manic-depressive retains an image of others as being either all good or all bad. The Washington group concluded that when such patients recognize others as separate, as being both good and bad, they experience a great deal of anxiety since this accurate view interferes with the needed idealization and dependency on others.

A last problem in therapy that is mentioned is communication. Manic-depressives were experienced as erecting barriers to true emotional interchange with others and displaying a lack of empathy. This problem appears to be a logical permutation of the patient's inordinate needs and his distortion of the other as all good and all-giving, so that the patient holds his feelings in check lest he offend the needed other. Such individuals also do not appear to want to discuss their underlying problems; rather, they utilize the sessions only to obtain reassurance. These therapeutic problems will be discussed more fully in chapters 9 and 13.

These two works of the Washington group on severely disturbed manic-depressive patients are extremely important in the psychoanalytic literature on depression. The authors objectively evaluated the family atmosphere, the early parent-child interactions, and the later experiences of the depressed individual, and related these events to the personality of the depressed patient and to his problems in treatment. They appreciated the significance of cultural and interpersonal factors as well as some of the internal dynamics of their patients and thus arrived at a more comprehensive view of the disorder.

Gibson (1958) replicated the study of the Washington group, using a questionnaire on the same patients. In comparing this group of manicdepressives with a group of schizophrenic patients, he found that the manic-depressives came from homes where there was greater pressure for achievement and prestige and a prevailing atmosphere of competitiveness and envy, and that manic-depressives showed greater concern for social acceptance. However, there is an overall paucity of family studies on depression, especially in comparison to the large number of investigations of family transactions in the genesis of schizophrenia. It appears paradoxical that while many theorists have stressed the importance of interpersonal relationships in depression, they have continued to focus on intrapsychic mechanisms in their research. On the other hand, although the pioneering studies of the Washington group are valuable, at times there seems to be an oversimplification of the depressive's inner life and a lack of appreciation of the complexity of internal psychodynamics.

The culturalist view of depression has stressed in its explanation of the disorder a reaction to social demands, the effect of the symptoms on others, and the use of depression to satisfy abnormal goals. Perhaps the first attempt at an analysis of depression from this standpoint was written by Alfred Adler as early as 1914. In a work entitled *Melancholie* (quoted in Ansbacher and Ansbacher 1956), Adler states that "Such individuals will always try to lean on others and will not scorn the use of exaggerated hints at their own inadequacy to force the support, adjustment, and submissiveness of others." Melancholics are said to suffer from an alleged "disability compensation." By this, Adler means that depressed individuals inflate the hazards of everyday life as they strive for unreachable lofty goals, and then blame others or life circumstances for the failure to achieve such goals. In the same work Adler states, "actually there is no psychological disease from which the environment suffers more and is more reminded of its unworthiness than melancholia." (Cited in Ansbacher and Ansbacher, 1956). In this manner the depressive displays both his anger at not getting his own way and his contempt for others. By debasing the world and exaggerating its perils, the depressive is said to compensate for his lack of desired yet unreasonable success.

Kurt Adler (1961) further stated the position of individual psychology (Alfred Adler's theoretical system) on depression, showing how this disorder fits into Adler's general theory of human behavior. According to the Adlerian school, psychopathology results from a striving for superiority which develops in order to compensate for feelings of inferiority. However, since these resultant grandiose aspirations rarely can be achieved, the individual develops a system of rationalizations or excuses to adjust to his imagined failures. These adopted alibis and evasions are both safeguarding maneuvers; they protect the self-esteem of the individual as well as the symptoms of a pathological mode of life. In depression, it is assumed that the individual has learned to exploit his weaknesses and complaints in order to force others to give him his way and thus to avoid life's responsibilities. By his self-bemoaning, the depressive forces others to comply with his wishes, extorting sympathy and making others sacrifice themselves for him. He is willing to go to any cost to prove to others how sick and disabled he is, and to escape from social obligations and reciprocal friendship.

The depressive's disdain for others, according to Adler, can be seen during his healthy interludes when his excessive ambition takes over and he reveals his ruthlessness and his unwillingness to exert effort to achieve results. When he fails, the depressive regularly blames others, his upbringing, ill fortune, or even his very depression.

Kurt Adler summarizes the depressive personality: "This then is the relentless effort of the depressed: To prevail with his will over others, to extort from them sacrifices, to frustrate all of their efforts to help him, to blame them—overtly or secretly—for his plight, and to be free of all social obligation and cooperations, by certifying to his sickness" (1961, p. 59).

In the current psychiatric literature, Bonime (1960, 1962, 1976) has been the most persuasive exponent of the culturalist position on depression. Bonime's contention is that depression is not simply a group of symptoms that make up a periodic illness, but that it is a *practice*, an everyday mode of interacting. Any interference with this type of functioning leads to an outward appearance of clinical depression in order to coerce the environment into letting the individual reinstate his usual interpersonal behaviors. The major pathological elements in this specific way of life are manipulativeness, aversion to influence by others, an unwillingness to give gratification, a basic sense of hostility, and the experience of anxiety.

By manipulativeness Bonime means the alleged dependency of the depressive, which is interpreted as a covert maneuver to exploit the generosity or responsibility of others. The depressive demands a response from others but gives nothing in return. In so doing, he deprives himself of true affection or fulfillment, striving only to have others do as he wishes. In proportion to his manipulativeness, the depressive is intolerant of influence from others and often misinterprets their genuine attempts to help him as the covert intention to control him. In a similar way Bonime asserts that the depressive refuses to acknowledge the responsibilities of life, subjectively sensing them as unfair demands.

Finally, Bonime interprets much of the depressive's outward behavior as disguised hostility. The depressive makes sure that others are affected by his suffering. Bonime finds themes of revenge and thus of anger to play a prominent role in the psyche of the depressionprone individual. The other major affective experience in depression is anxiety which is experienced when others are unresponsive to the patient's usual machinations. However, the depressive quite often overcomes this anxiety by shifting his manipulative style and regaining his effectiveness. This anxiety is "primarily a sense of the threat of failing to function effectively as a depressive" (1976, p. 318).

Bonime believes that the etiology of adult depression can be found in a childhood that lacked the needed nurturance and respect from parents. Instead, the child's true emotional needs were ignored or squelched so that he grew up feeling he had been cheated and solicitude was still due from others. To quote Bonime, "Despite the wide variety of depression-prone individuals, however, a constant underlying dynamic factor in their personalities is the grim pursuit of the unrealized (or incompletely realized) childhood" (1976, p. 321).

Other psychoanalytic authors such as

Chodoff (1970), Salzman and Masserman (1962), and Saperstein and Kaufman (1966) have also made contributions that stress the social rather than instinctual or libidinal roots of depression. Their emphasis has also been on the interpersonal aspects of the disorder as well as on the depressive's unrealistic yet desperately needed personal goals (and the appearance of clinical depression either when interpersonal responsiveness is not elicited or when there is a failure to achieve the grandiose goals). Becker (1964) has proposed an intriguing theory that contrasts the social consequences of depression and schizophrenia. According to Becker, schizophrenia demonstrates a disregard for social conventions, and depression represents an over-trained individual who conforms too strongly to cultural values but needs these stringent guidelines for his sense of well-being.

Becker also speculates that the depressive limits his object ties to only a few individuals, so that losing one of these object ties hits him especially hard. The depressive is conceptualized as going through a monotonous repetition of behavior for the approval of a select few. Becker writes, "In our culture we are familiar with the person who lives his life for the wishes of his parents and becomes depressed when they die and he has reached the age of forty or fifty. He has lost the only audience for whom the plot in which he was performing was valid. He is left in the hopeless despair of the actor who knows only one set of lines, and loses the one audience who wants to hear it" (1964, p. 127).

Whether Adler's thesis of depression as power through illness, or Bonime's view of depression as obstinacy and refusal to accept social responsibility, or Becker's exposition of depression as over-conformity is accepted, it cannot be doubted that the culturalist tradition has enriched the understanding of this disorder by demonstrating how it intermeshes with cultural expectations and social relationships. The culturalist sees depression as part of the fabric of sociocultural intercourse, and not as an isolated phenomenon. At the same time there is a relative lack of appreciation for depression as a personal experience, or of how the patient actually suffers in his melancholic sorrow. So much attention is given to what the depressive wishes to achieve, evade, or manipulate that one senses that the actual individual and his inner life have been overlooked. The interpersonal and culturalist orientations have served as significant correctives to the excessive concern for the internal dynamics that the early psychoanalytic writers had with depression. However, they often appear equally limited in their zeal to point out the external aspects of depression as the very "internally oriented" theorists that they criticize.

The Existentialist School

This approach to psychopathology has received only limited exposure in the United States, perhaps because it utilizes its own peculiar terminology and is based largely on continental philosophical schools which are quite complex and foreign to the training of most American psychotherapists. Stated very briefly, the task of the existentialist student of psychopathology is to describe the phenomenological world of the patient without recourse to excessive nonexperiential concepts (such as unconscious dynamics) or selected causal events (such as heredity or childhood traumas). Existential or phenomenologic analysis is the examination of the world as it is grasped intuitively by an active consciousness, without any preconceived structures. Karl Jaspers (1964) has written a massive work in which he discusses all of psychopathology from this point of view. He starts by making "some representation of what is really happening in our patients, what they are actually going through, how it strikes them, how they feel." Then he progresses to the establishment of meaningful connections between experiences, and culminates in an encompassing of the patient in his total being as revealed through the patient's experience.

Minkowski (1958) reported a case of "schizophrenic depression" from this standpoint and concluded that his patient's melancholic delusions logically derived from a distorted sense of time. Arieti (1974) summarizes other existential studies by Le Mappian, Ey, and Sommer as interpreting the condition to be an arrest or insufficiency of all vital activities. There is said to be a "pathetic immobility, a suspension of existence, a syncope of time" according to Ey (cited in Arieti, 1974). These authors also stress the importance of time distortion in the experience of depression; there is an excessive concern with past events which are constantly in mind and which the individual uses to torture himself with guilty recriminations. Beck (1967) summarizes a large study by Tellenbach on the analysis of the case histories of   140

melancholics. Tellenbach found that the world of the depressive is dominated by orderliness, conscientiousness, and an overriding need to please significant others. These patients are further reported as seeking security and avoiding situations which might elicit guilt. Paradoxically, this overconscientiousness often leads the patient to feel obliged to place impossibly exacting demands on himself in order to escape guilt. When the demands simply cannot be fulfilled, clinical depression may ensue. Perhaps the most famous existential studies, however, concern not depression but mania. Binswanger (1933) investigated the inner experience of the manic patient. He concluded that logic is abandoned and difficulties diminished, and life exists only for the concrete moment. The "Ideenflucht," or flight of ideas, reveals that language ceases to be used for communication but rather becomes a source of play and fun. Distortions of time and space also are noted in the manic.

Sullivan, who was certainly not of the existential school, gives a remarkably clinical and almost phenomenologic description of depression (1940, p. 102). He mentions the stereotyped, repetitive tendency toward destructive situations, the preoccupation with a limited number of ideas, and the retardation of vital processes. He further believed that relating the onset of depression to a publicly understandable cause was merely a way of rationalizing one's suffering and of "integrating the experience into the self without loss of prestige and uncertainty about (his) social and personal future" (1940, p. 105). Thus Sullivan appears to dismiss the premise that depressions are reactions to life events.

These studies were partially a reaction to the traditional psychoanalytic neglect of the individual's actual conscious experience for the intricacies of unconscious drives and dynamics, although they also may be seen as psychiatric applications of Heidegger's basic existential philosophy.[6]

The existentialists allow us a more detailed and accurate picture of the subjective world of the individual. In this significant manner, existential studies complement the understanding derived by the other psychoanalytic approaches. Despite the extent to which one agrees with their basic philosophy, these studies are worth reading for their vivid and penetrating accounts of how the disorder affects the patient's conscious life.

Beck's Cognitive Theory

Since the earliest description of depressive illness, distortions in cognition, such as extreme pessimism or unrealistic self-reproaches, have been noted by most authors as part of the symptom complex. The originality of Beck's view is that he considers these cognitive distortions to be the primary cause of the disorder rather than secondary elaborations. According to Beck, all forms of psychopathology (not just schizophrenia) manifest thought disorder to some degree. Obviously no one can know reality in a completely objective way, and each person's appreciation of his world is colored by his past experiences. Therefore, so-called reality testing must remain a largely subjective affair. However, there is usually consensual agreement on most experiences and, since this agreement is shared by the overwhelming majority, such perspectives are considered to be within the normal range. In psychopathology, according to Beck, characteristic distortions appear that deviate from what most individuals would consider a realistic mode of thinking or of interpreting reality.

Depression presents its own specific types of distortion which Beck has labeled the "cognitive triad" (1970). This consists of

1. negative expectations of the environment

2. a negative view of oneself 3. negative expectations of the future

Beck states that he was able to trace these core elements of depression from his patients' dreams, free associations, and reactions to external stimuli. He also presents extensive experimental data, usually obtained by depression inventory scales, to support his conclusions (Beck, 1967).

Most students of depression would agree that depressed patients often have pessimistic views regarding others, themselves, and their future. The difficulty arises when cognition is considered to be primary, and as giving rise to the affect of depression. For Beck, appropriate feelings of depression would spontaneously arise out of this cognitive stance, although he does not explain how. In a more recent work (1976) Beck relates depression to a significant loss, which in turn gives rise to the characteristic cognitive distortions. Beck writes that "the patient's experiences in living thus activate cognitive patterns revolving around the theme of loss. The various emotional, motivational, behavioral, and vegetative phenomena of depression flow from these negative self-evaluations" (1976, p. 129).

Beck continues patient's sadness is an inevitable consequence of his sense of deprivation, pessimism, and self-criticism" (1976, 129). He concludes that experiencing loss "after (either as the result of an

actual, obvious event or insidious deprivations) the depression-prone person begins to appraise his experiences in a negative way" (1976, p. 129).

Beck has produced a tremendous amount of clinical and experimental work documenting his particular theory. Although it has great merit, his formulation also suffers from some drawbacks. Beck undoubtedly has done psychiatry a service by emphasizing the cognitive aspects of depression. However, he has focused on mainly conscious and simple cognitive formulations. He ignores the significant role of unconscious cognitive structures, as well as the role of conflict. For example, some depressives harbor expectations which doom them to disappointment and despair, yet these expectations are unconscious and the individual is unaware of the influence they exert on his behavior. Similarly, other depressives are ashamed of their unrealistic dependency needs or irrational ambitions and actively fight against these unpleasant aspects of the self. This area of conflict is neglected by Beck, so at times his theory of depression smacks of only "wrong thinking" and does not do justice to the complexity of the human psyche.

Beck's theory is also weak in determining why certain people become depressed following a loss and others do not. He does not really consider the interpersonal aspects of the depression-prone person and why a loss or disappointment precipitates a depressive episode. He merely relates that a loss sets off a self-reinforcing chain reaction which culminates in depression. The depressed person is described as "regarding himself as lacking some element or attribute that he considers essential for his happiness" (1976, p. 105). However, why this should lead to the "cognitive triad" is not fully explained.

Beck actually describes the results but not the cause of depression. He offers a version of depression only in cross-section, not in its longitudinal and psychodynamic unfolding. He states that upon clinical recovery the individual no longer distorts his experiences; yet the basic personality has not changed. Therefore, although Beck quite accurately describes some of the cognitive distortions seen during a depressive episode, he does not appear to go beyond these conscious beliefs to the underlying—often unconscious, conflictual, or interpersonal— patterns that make the individual vulnerable to depression in the first place.

In spite of these limitations, Beck's work is exemplary and points the way to the neglected area of cognition in psychopathology. His influence in the field is well deserved.

Seligman's Learned Helplessness Model

In experiments involving the administration of inescapable shock to dogs, Seligman and his colleagues (Seligman and Maier, 1967) discovered a reaction which they termed "learned helplessness." They found that after exposing dogs to a series of painful stimuli in a situation that prevented escape, the animals did not avoid the painful stimuli even when escape was possible. It appeared that the dogs had given up and had learned to endure helplessly the painful shocks. Seligman generalized these findings to human depression: he suggested that the depressive has been blocked from mastering adaptive techniques to deal with painful situations, instead learning helplessness. At the core of this theory is the hypothesis that the depressive sees no relationship between his responses and the reinforcement he receives from the environment. Experience with repeated trials, in which the individual eventually found that his efforts made no difference in terms of reward, caused this set of learned behaviors to become generalized and internalized into a personality trait.

Therefore Seligman asserts that the depressive has a history characterized by failure to control environmental rewards. Depression ensues when the individual feels he has lost all control over environmental responses and, due to his learned helplessness, perceives himself as unable to alter this ungratifying state of affairs.

He then falls into a state of passivity, misery, and hopelessness. He believes that his behavior lacks meaning because it is so ineffective in bringing about reinforcement. It is important to stress that in contrast to Beck, Seligman differentiates overall negative expectations from learned helplessness. He states that "according to our model, depression is not generalized pessimism but pessimism specific to the effects of one's own skilled actions" (1975, p. 86). Furthermore, he does not believe that his model can account for all affective disorders but only those "in which the individual is slow to initiate responses, believes himself to be powerless and hopeless, and sees his future as bleak..." (1975, p. 81). Seligman's model has much to recommend it in that it is an empirical hypothesis that lends itself to direct experimental confirmation (Miller and Seligman, 1976).

While Seligman is correct in describing many depressives as feeling helpless to control environmental reinforcement, this situation is only part of the total depressive picture. Some authors such as Adler and Bonime view the actual depressive episode as the depressive's attempt to force the environment to fulfill his needs, so that he is far from helpless. According to this view, proclaimed helplessness is a devious manipulation to force others to give the depressive what he wants. Even without entertaining this concept of depression, there are some difficulties with the "learned helplessness" model. Many depressives seek to reinstate the lost sources of pleasure by hard work, selfdenial, or guilt-inducing behavior. Therefore the depressive is not helpless; rather, he has learned specific ways—however inappropriate—to gain the reinforcement he requires. The vulnerability of the depressive appears to reside in his inordinate need of external reinforcement for self-esteem or well-being, rather than in his not knowing how to get the needed reinforcement. Depressives are too reliant on external sources for achieving a sense of meaning in their lives, and therefore they become very skilled at elaborating interpersonal maneuvers to keep the needed relationships in an ongoing state.

If they happen to lose the external sources of gratification, then they manifest helplessness in terms of deriving meaning from life or in their ability to derive reinforcement from self-directed activities. It is not that the depressive sees no connection between response and reinforcement, but that his system of reinforcement may be too precarious and limited.

It appears that Seligman has taken the results of a depressive episode to be its cause. During a depressive attack the individual may bemoan his fate, take no initiative on his own behalf, and appear totally helpless. However, this clinical picture may be part of the depressive's characteristic tendency to have others supply meaning and gratification for him. When these external sources are removed either through loss or through another's inability to comply with his manipulations, the depressive may indeed feel that he cannot reinstate the needed external sources of gratification by direct action. However, this pattern is not a result of learned helplessness, which assumes no perceived connection between response and reinforcement. Rather, as mentioned previously, it may be the result of an excessive reliance on external others or on the achievement of an external goal from which to derive meaning and gratification. Depressives do have selfinhibitions in certain crucial areas (to be dealt with in chapters 6 and 7), but their areas of inhibition are not a result of a lack of reward for effort, as Seligman's model suggests.

Physiological Approaches

This book is not intended to be an authoritative and detailed text on organic theories of depression, nor do I claim any firsthand experience with research on this aspect of depression. However, in order to give a more complete view of approaches to depression, some of the major physiological theories are briefly outlined below.

Before describing these theories, it should be clarified that a physiological approach to depression does not necessarily contradict a psychodynamic approach. Certainly, neurological events accompany psychological phenomena, and the experience of depression is no exception. The two views are particularly congruent if depression is conceptualized as a basic affect that automatically arises in certain situations, as exemplified in the theories of Sandler and Joffe (1965) and Bibring (1953). The more complex view of depression as being the result of complicated metapsychological events does not lend itself so easily to concordance with biochemical approaches, since according to this conceptualization depression may be further reduced to basic drives or structures. Therefore biochemical theories favor a view of depression as a basic emotion (see chapter 7) having both psychological and physiological correlates.

The modern biochemical view of depression came about as a result of a series of serendipitous clinical observations that later were backed up with animal research studies. In the early 1950s, it was found that some hypertensive patients treated with reserpine developed episodes of depression. Reserpine has been shown to deplete the brain of norepinephrine (NE) and serotonin or 5hydroxytryptamine (5-HT). At the same time, in another study clinicians noted that some tubercular patients treated with isoniazid showed unexpected elevations of mood. Isoniazid has been shown to block the destruction of NE and 5-HT by inhibiting the effect of monoamine oxidase (MAO), an enzyme that metabolizes these amines. It was further discovered in animal research studies that other compounds which blocked the action of MAO could reverse the depression-like syndrome caused by reserpine. The beneficial effects of tricyclic antidepressants such as imipramine were eventually shown by Hertting (Prange, 1973) to result from a blockage of the re-uptake of NE at nerve endings. Lithium, a drug effective in decreasing mania, in contrast was believed to enhance the re-uptake of NE at the synaptic cleft.

These clinical observations and the subsequent imposing research have singled out these two compounds, NE and 5-HT, as specifically related to depression. These amines are believed to be neurotransmitters; that is, they conduct excitation from one neurone on another. It has been postulated that an excess of either one or both of these amines leads to mania, and a depletion leads to depression.

The metabolic pathways for NE and 5-HT are presented in Table 2-1 (Akiskal and McKinney, 1975).

Table 2-1

The metabolic pathways for NE and 5-HT

Amino Acid Precursor	Active Amine	Metabolite
Tyrosine——Dopamine (DA)——	Norepinephrine——	3-Methoxy-4-Hydroxy phenelethylene Glycol (MHPG)
		Homovanillic Acid (HVA)
L-Tryptophan—5-Hydroxytryptophan—Serotonin (5-HT)——		5-Hydroxy indoleacetic Acid (5-HIAA)

In the United States NE has been selected as

the active amine, while in Europe attention has been given to serotonin (5-HT) as the neurotransmitter implicated in depression. The success of drugs that alter the levels of these amines in the brain in treating depressive episodes has led to a great deal of study and even the hope that eventually the various subtypes of depression may be differentiated by biochemical tests alone (Schildkraut, 1975).

Support for the "indoleamine hypothesis," which implicates a decrease of 5-HT as the active compound in depressive disorders, has come from a series of studies. The best known are those of Coppen and his colleagues (1963), in which tryptophan, a precursor of 5-HT, was shown to potentiate the antidepressant effect of an MAO inhibitor. It was reasoned that the greater antidepressant effect was due to an increased level of 5-IIT. However, similar results have not been found in repeated studies (Mendels, 1974). The antidepressant effect of tryptophan alone also has not been shown uniformly (Goodwin and Bunney, 1973).

Other evidence that supports the serotonindepletion hypothesis has been the finding of lower than normal concentrations of 5-HIAA, a metabolite of serotonin, both in the cerebrospinal fluid of depressed patients and in the brain tissue of suicide victims (Bunney et al., 1972).

Studies that do not support the role of 5-IIT in affective disorders involve the failure to produce depression by drugs that block the synthesis of serotonin. Patients with carcinoid syndrome who were given the drug parachlorophenylalanine (PCPA) displayed a variety of psychic abnormalities such as anxiety, irritability, or negativism, but not depression. The same drug even at high doses also had little effect when administered to monkeys (Redmond et al., 1971). Therefore, depletion of 5-HT by itself does not appear to result in depression, although this amine still is believed to play a role in the biochemistry of affective disorders in combination with other physiological alterations.

The other major biochemical hypothesis involves the brain catecholamine NE, and its precursor, dopamine (DA). The major exponent of this hypothesis is Schildkraut, who periodically has reviewed the pertinent literature (1965, 1975; Durell and Schildkraut, 1966) in addition to contributing many research and clinical studies. As with serotonin, researchers have found decreased levels of NE in the urine of some but not all depressed patients. In one study done by Schinfecker in 1965 (cited in Schildkraut, 1975) a regular cycle of NE metabolite excretion was found to correlate with the phases of mania and depression in cyclothymic patients; high NE excretion started with the onset of a manic phase and low NE excretion reflected the depressive phase. Again, the theory postulates that a depletion of NE (as caused by reserpine) results in depression, a restoration of adequate brain NE-levels (as a result of tricyclic antidepressants or MAO inhibitors) relieves the depression, and an excess of NE is responsible for mania.

Schildkraut cites numerous studies in support of this hypothesis, but he also mentions a great deal of data that question the theory. Among the contradictory findings are the following: (1) catecholamine excretion is not lowered in all depressed patients, but mainly in agitated or anxious individuals; (2) the concentration of plasma catecholamines was found to be much more correlated with anxiety than depression. Therefore muscular activity (in mania, anxiety states, or agitated depression) may be the cause of NE excretion levels rather than depression itself. Another difficulty is that urinary NE reflects total body reactions and may not be considered a reliable reflection of brain catecholamine metabolism.

It has recently been suggested that MHPG, a metabolite of NE that is found in the urine, may parallel the levels of brain NE and only partially reflect body levels of catecholamines (Schildkraut, 1975). Initial studies with MHPG have shown a correlation with mood, but once again, contradictory findings have also been reported. Variations in MHPG excretion in response to general stress (not just affective disorders) have been reported, so its specific relationship to depression and mania remains to be established. Finally, not all depressed patients show low excretion of MHPG. This last finding has suggested that there may be different biochemical types of depression that vary in response to certain drugs.

Mendels (1975) found no noticeable improvement in depressed patients who were given large doses of L-Dopa, the immediate precursor of DA. This L-Dopa dosage should have increased the brain levels of DA and also perhaps NE. As with serotonin, most researchers believe that catecholamines are somehow related to affective disorders but that these amines are only part of a very complex metabolic process that has yet to be elucidated.

While the beneficial effects of the tricyclic antidepressants and of the MAO inhibitors have greatly helped in the treatment of depression, attempts to correlate these clinical effects into a comprehensive biochemical theory have not been successful as yet. Reviews of experimental work (Akiskal and McKinney, 1975; Baldessarini, 1975; Goodwin and Bunney, 1973) all agree that these amines somehow are implicated in affective disorders but that there is still insufficient knowledge of brain biochemistry to make conclusive statements. That the proposed model of affective disorders entails a direct reflection of the levels of biogenic amines in the brain has been recognized as too simplistic by most investigators.

Some of the objections to this model have been discussed by Baldessarini (1975) in an excellent review article and they will be noted briefly here. Baldessarini argues that so-called animal depressions, which are induced by drugs on which much of the biochemical theories depend, actually bear little resemblance to naturally occurring depression in humans. Rather, the reserpine-induced "depression" in monkeys resembles a state of sedation. In fact, the drugs which best reverse these animal "depressions," L-Dopa and amphetamines, have the least clinical effect on human depression. Baldessarini further argues that reserpine depression may not be at all typical of human depression, for it has been found that the effects of this drug are highly variable in different individuals; some respond with lethargy, others with an organic brain syndrome, and others with no mental changes. Those individuals who became depressed after taking reserpine had a previous history of depression and thus may have been predisposed to react with depression by past experience.

Another criticism of drug research strategy is that most experiments study only the immediate biochemical effects of drugs rather than their chronic effects over time. This may be especially misleading in affective disorders since there is a considerable lag in clinical response to most antidepressant medications. The fact of therapeutic response lag after drug ingestion has led Mandell and Segal (1975) to postulate a theory of depression that is almost an exact reverse of the catecholamine hypothesis. They believe that depression may be due to an excess of brain catecholamine activity and that antidepressant drugs, by increasing the level of catecholamines, affect the enzymes and other macromolecules which synthesize catecholamines. These drugs would cause a decrease of natural production of catecholamines because the enzymes would adapt to the high levels of amines from the drugs. Since this adaptive process would require several days, they assume that their theory fits the clinical data better. The biochemical cause of affective disorders would reside in a general biochemical system that controls the levels and types of neurotransmitters in significant parts of the brain, rather than residing in the periodic excess of any catecholamine. This provocative hypothesis is far from being proven, although Mandell and Segal cite Oswald's (1972) study in which normals receiving antidepressants reported an initial discomfort, presumably due to an excess of catecholamines. However, depressed patients who receive similar drugs do not report an initial exacerbation of their symptoms.

The further significance of Mandell and Segal's work is that it points out that antidepressant drugs have many biochemical actions and may affect many systems other than biogenic amine levels. These other systems may ultimately be responsible for clinical effects of antidepressant drugs. This view is further borne out by the lack of absolute correlation between clinical response and catecholamine or indoleamine levels. The difficulties with accepting a simple model of biogenic amine levels as responsible for depression solely because antidepressants appear to affect the levels of these compounds is well summarized by Baldessarini (1975).

"There may be a risk of a *post hoc, ergo propter hoc* logical fallacy in this field, as it is often accepted uncritically that responsiveness of a behavioral disorder to a physical therapy implies not only the existence of an organicmetabolic cause, but furthermore that the cause involves metabolic changes opposite to those produced by treatment. This conclusion is no more logical than the proposition that a careful study of the pharmacology of the clinically effective preparations of Foxglove, Squill, or Mercury would have disclosed information of fundamental importance to the etiology of dropsy." (p. 1092)

While the most heuristic and prominent physiological approach to depression has involved biogenic amines, other biological systems have been investigated and may be briefly mentioned. For a long time, endocrine changes were felt to be involved with affective disorders since depression or elation may accompany some endocrinopathies. Some studies had shown a correlation between the excretion of 17-hydroxycortico-steroids and changes in affective disorders (Gibbons, 1967), while other researchers found no such relationship (Kurland, 1964). In a carefully controlled study, Sachar et al. (1972) observed that cortisol production was greatly affected by emotional arousal, anxiety, or psychotic decompensation, but not by depression itself. Apathetic depressed individuals showed no changes in adrenocortical activity during or after their depressive episodes. From this study, and from the contradictory data of other studies, it may be tentatively assumed that cortisol levels reflect the general state of upset of an individual, independent of affective disorders.

The other endocrine system implicated in depression is the thyroid-pituitary axis. Prange et al. (1969) found that l-tri-iodothyronine enhanced the effect of imipramine in depressed females. In a later study Prange and Wilson (1972) found that thyrotropin-releasing hormone by itself may be an effective antidepressant. However, Prange relates this therapeutic result to an effect on catecholamine metabolism that is independent of thyroid functioning. In fact, although Prange has utilized thyroid-related substances in his clinical research, he is an adherent of the so-called biogenic amine "permissive hypothesis," which postulates an initial serotonin deficiency that makes an individual susceptible to depression when NE levels are low, or mania when NE levels are high (Prange, 1973). Therefore the endocrine system does not at present appear to be a promising area of research in the affective disorders.

The other major area of biochemical interest has to do with membrane transport and electrolyte balance. This line of investigation has been greatly stimulated by the success of lithium, a simple alkali metal (like sodium and potassium) used in treating acute manic attacks (Cade, 1949). Later, lithium was used as a prophylaxis for manic-depression (Baastrup and Schou, 1967) and more recently it has been tried in patients who have recurrent depression without the presence of mania (Fieve et al., 1968).

Once again the successful employment of a drug has understandably led to speculations about the nature of the illness based on the biochemical effect of the drug. In the case of lithium, it was noted that there was an initial loss of sodium which was followed after a few days by compensatory sodium retention in some patients (Tupin, 1972). It is not clear whether this effect on sodium by lithium occurs at the cellular level or through a mediating action of aldosterone (Aronoff et al., 1971).

Some investigators believe that lithium alters the ionic concentration of sodium and potassium at the cell membranes of neurones, retards neuronal transmission, and thus "slows down" the manic patient. This hypothesis is questionable since lithium also has been effective in some forms of depression. Others

(Greenspan et al., 1970; Messina et al., 1970) have attempted to relate lithium administration to alterations in catecholamine metabolism. At present this area of research is too new to have crystallized a major synthesizing hypothesis. Lithium studies remain an extremely actively pursued avenue of investigation in the biochemistry of affective disorders.

This very brief review of physiological approaches to depression and mania is intended to present some basic and unfortunately limited information about this fertile approach to affective disorders which is usually ignored by psychotherapists. It was stressed at the beginning of this section that a physiological approach to depression need not contradict a psychodynamic view if depression is conceived to be a basic affect. It is unfortunate that the study of mental illness too often has become split into warring camps of organically and psychologically oriented practitioners. Obviously the clinician cannot ignore the fact that there are biological events occurring in the brain of the patient any more than the chemical researcher can ignore that the substances he is studying are affected by the life experiences of the organism.

Summary

Over the years, theories of depression have reflected the prevailing climate of psychoanalysis. It may be observed that the recent theories (with notable exceptions) have relied less on metapsychology and have grown closer to clinical experience. Modern theories of depression appear less speculative even if less imaginative. Similarly, an appreciation of cultural and interpersonal factors has become noticeable as psychoanalysis has moved away from an instinctual, mainly hydraulic model to a more encompassing theory that no longer seeks to reduce all behavior to unconscious transformations of energy. Certainly, the political and social milieu as well as changes in basic scientific theory have influenced the evolution of psychoanalytic thought, which in turn has affected the conceptualization of depression.

The psychoanalytic inquiry into depression has not been without critics and some evaluation appears justified. In a recent review article, Chodoff (1972) rightly mentions that in many contributions the current degree of the patient's illness, from which observations have been generalized, is not specified. For example, Freud clearly indicated that his formulations were intended only to apply to very disturbed melancholics. Yet others have applied his theory to less impaired individuals or they have not bothered to specify the degree of impairment of the patients that they described. Chodoff also believes that too much of the literature has been influenced by the study of manic-depressive psychosis, with a relative neglect of other varieties of depression.

Another criticism is that the contributors to the psychoanalytic literature on depression based their findings on the intensive analysis of only a few individuals and the size of their sample was too small for generalizations. Unfortunately, it is one of the limitations of the psychoanalytic method; that each practitioner can only treat a limited number of individuals on so intense a level in his lifetime. Yet this is the traditional model of clinical medicine where a series of patients with a similar condition is reported, and the similarities and differences noted. Larger experimental studies may utilize a greater number of patients, but at the cost of achieving what are mainly common-sense and pedestrian findings. Chodoff (1972) has also noted this limitation of nonpsychoanalytic studies, stating that their level of observation is often superficial. He believes that psychoanalytic investigations are far more intensive and searching, but that in contrast to more scientifically controlled studies, there is sometimes a confusion between observed and inferred material. Another scientific criticism leveled at psychodynamic reports is that there is a failure to utilize a control group. This criticism does not appear to carry too much weight since it is assumed that the other nondepressed patients in the analysts' practices are sufficiently different (in that they are not included in the description of depressed individuals) to serve as a nonreported but nonetheless existent control group.

A more telling limitation of psychodynamic studies may be the repeated tendency of authors to fit depression into a pre-existing general theory of psychopathology. The more general theory at times seems like a pro-crustean bed that allows only those features of depression that fit the theory to be considered, while distorting or ignoring other aspects that may contradict the basic formulations. This does appear to be a failing of many of the theories, and their specific biases have been mentioned along with their positive contributions. It may be best to view the formulations of each school as a different perspective on a uniform clinical problem, with each viewpoint complementing the others and highlighting important constructs that have been omitted by others. The Freudians, the Kleinians, the interpersonal theorists, and all the others we have considered here have contributed to our understanding of depression, and as much as possible their work should be considered as a totality.

While the differences in the theory may be seen as changes in the psychoanalytic Zeitgeist, it is also possible that the clinical nature of depression itself has changed over the decades. The guilty, paralyzed melancholics described in the early literature are seen infrequently today. Rather, most depressions appear to be milder, with less self-recriminations and more of a demanding quality motivated by thwarted aspirations. It may be that as society becomes less rigidly moralistic, and as childhood upbringing becomes more permissive, the superficial aspects of the syndrome may change. Similarly, the greater mobility between social and economic classes may promote more pressure for achievement than in a static, controlled caste society. Therefore the differences in the theories presented may accurately reflect changes in the type of patient seen.

Finally there is the real possibility that depression may result from different causes in different individuals. Depression may well be the final common pathway for various processes that alter the psychological equilibrium in different patients. Not all depressives may be alike, although, as with any scientific inquiry, the goal of the investigator is to search behind clinical differences to find basic, general principles at a higher level of inference from which the symptomatic picture may logically be deduced. Despite the disparity of theoretical systems, it cannot have escaped the reader's attention that certain basic themes have occurred again and again. Therefore, even while starting from vastly different philosophical beliefs about the nature of psychopathology, most authors have noted specific core features in depressed individuals.

Before closing this chapter, it should be noted that the authors of this book have made some contributions of their own toward an understanding of depression. These works have not been included in this review because a fuller exposition of our views will be presented in later chapters. It is hoped that this cursory tour through the history of the concept of melancholia will provide a foundation for the more detailed material to follow, and help to place it in proper perspective.

Notes

[1] The reader is referred to the excellent reviews by Lewis (1934), Jellife (1931), and Zilboorg (1941) for a more exhaustive account of the early psychiatric studies of depression.

[2] It may be of interest that Freud criticized Abraham as placing too much importance on libidinal stages and ignoring the other aspects of the personality. (See Jones, 1955. Vol. II.)

[3] At this point, this judgmental part of the ego is called the conscience but clearly it later becomes the superego with the revision brought about by the structural theory.

[4] An interesting historical finding is that in 1920 George Carver, an English psychiatrist, independently arrived at conclusions very similar to those espoused by Freud in an analysis of a depressed patient. Carver emphasized his patient's unconscious anger against her dead husband for having abandoned her, but went on further to speak of an "identification of the self with a beloved person who is blamed for having caused the deprivation." Carver wrote that the major mechanism in the case "seems to be a displacement of the reproach from the environment including the husband, to the self; analysis showing th abuse which the patient heaped so lavishly upon hersel was really intended for the former" (Carver, 1921; cited in Mendelson, 1974).

[5] The interested reader may find a summary of Klein's system in Hannah Segal's excellent book (1964).

[6] Binswanger's concise paper "Heidegger's Analytic of Existence and Its Meaning for Psychiatry" (1963) is an excellent statement of the existentialist position and is recommended as an introduction for the interested reader.

THE MANIFEST SYMPTOMATOLOGY OF DEPRESSION IN ADULTS

Silvano Arieti

Introductory Remarks and Classificatory Criteria

The manifest symptomatology of the various depressive syndromes requires careful examination and evaluation. Nevertheless, even more than in the study of other psychiatric conditions, an approach confined to the observation and assessment of the manifest symptomatology of depressions leaves the clinician with an awareness of the limitation of the method. The psychotherapist senses the profundity of the syndrome with which he deals, realizes that he cannot go far with a surface investigation, and feels the need for a psychodynamic approach. This in fact will be the procedure followed in this book.

The manifest symptomatology of depression

impresses the clinician as being relatively uniform, characterized at least in the majority of cases by one prevailing feature—the depressive mood. It does not present a multifaceted picture, leading to different sorts of inquiries, like that of the schizophrenic disorder. Contrary to the schizophrenic syndrome, it does not confront the therapist with an image so different from the usual one of the human being, and so distorted. However, it does have an especially powerful impact on the clinician who is struck by the intensity of the sorrow that he witnesses and to which he immediately responds with a sense of affinity, so close is that image of sorrow to a common part of the human condition. Moreover the clinical picture has a few important secondary traits which are often overlooked in the context of the mood of depression. Any description of the manifest symptomatology of the syndromes included under the category of depression implies some agreement on the classification of these syndromes. But such agreement has never been reached, since some aspects of these conditions are far from being clarified and several others are controversial. Some features which at our stage of knowledge seem to be fundamental marks of distinction may be proved later to be not so basic.

Any classification and description which are based on partial knowledge tend to repeat traditional ways, established by previous generations of professionals working in the field.

At the present level of our understanding the following three questions seem of pivotal importance in classificatory attempts.

Is the depression primary or secondary? A depression is called primary when it constitutes an important and/or essential component of a syndrome; for instance, in what is generally called "psychotic depression" or "severe depression."

In manic-depressive psychosis the depression is also primary. In fact, although the syndrome may have manic attacks, the depression is an important and probably necessary component. We say probably and not absolutely necessary because there are rare cases of the illness characterized only by manic attacks. In these cases, however, the presumptive evidence is that the depressive attacks occur at a subclinical or subliminal level.

A depression which occurs in the course of epilepsy or an endocrine syndrome is not considered primary because the available evidence suggests that it would not have occurred in the absence of the original syndrome.

Is the depression severe or mild? At times this question is formulated with different terminology: Is the depression endogenous or reactive; or, is the depression psychotic or neurotic? These terminologies reflect the theoretical premises of the persons who use them. An endogenous depression is based exclusively on organic, presumably hereditary factors which manifest themselves in biochemical alterations of the organism. A reactive depression would be one which is precipitated by an event perceived by the patient as harmful or unpleasant.

This dichotomy is not substantiated by any sure evidence. Any depression must ultimately be mediated by a living organism, and therefore it requires neurophysiological mechanisms and biochemical changes. On the other hand, we are not justified in claiming that no precipitating events exist just because we have not been able to determine them. In all depressions there are both psychological and biological, nonpsychological components. Moreover the biological components may not necessarily be based on anatomical pathology, but may be functional. In other words, they consist only of changes in some functions of the organism, but not of anatomical structures.

The authors of this book believe that in most cases it is possible to recognize whether a depression is psychotic or neurotic. However, these two terms have come to be used in incorrect ways by many authors and clinicians. They are wrongly used when a depression is called psychotic only if some symptoms are present which occur also in schizophrenia and are acknowledged by everybody as psychotic; for instance, hallucinations, delusions, or ideas of reference. These symptoms are not specific for any type of depression or for manic-depressive psychosis. The issue here hinges on the definition of psychosis.

As I wrote elsewhere (1973, 1974), psychosis is a term used by many to designate a severe or major psychiatric disorder. In theory and clinical practice the concept is more difficult to define because severity is not an inflexible characteristic. A certain number of cases diagnosed as psychosis may in fact be less serious from the point of view of the sufferer or of society than some cases included in other psychiatric categories. The term *psychosis* is at times indistinctly equated with insanity. The latter term, when used legally or in popular language, suggests a person who is so incompetent that he may require special control or supervision. However, psychosis indicates not only actual or potential severity, it also connotes that an unrealistic way of appreciating the self and the world is accepted and tends to be accepted by the sufferer as a normal way of living. This definition of psychosis lends itself to justified criticism because it implies that we know what is reality and what is unreality. Many philosophers would promptly indicate to us how naive we are in assuming that we have such knowledge.

In practical terms we can say that no matter what transformation the psychotic patient has undergone, that transformation becomes his way of relating to himself and to others and of interpreting the world. The organic psychotic patient has a cognitive defect but believes that the way he deals with the world is not defective. The schizophrenic undergoes predominantly a symbolic transformation, but he believes there is nothing wrong in living in accordance with that symbolic transformation.

The patient who is depressed to a psychotic degree has undergone predominantly a severe emotional transformation, but he believes that his way of feeling is appropriate to the circumstances in which he lives. Thus he does not fight his disorder, as the psychoneurotic does, but lives within it. In many cases he even seems to nourish it. In this respect he resembles persons who are affected by character neuroses and do not even know the pathological nature of their difficulties. The distortions of the character neuroses, however, are susceptible to at least partial adaptation to the demands of society, whereas in psychoses such adaptation is impossible or very difficult.

The severely depressed person may neglect feeding himself to the point of starvation; he may be so inactive as to be unable to take care of even the most elementary needs; he may think he is justified in believing that there is nothing good in life and death is preferable. He also considers any attempt to improve his life to be worthless, and in some cases he feels guilty in the absence of reasons which would make other people feel guilty. He may actually attempt suicide if he has an opportunity to implement such a plan. He considers his mood consonant with what appears to him the reality of his situation. Thus he seems to have characteristics which would make appropriate the designation "psychotic." Only in a minority of cases do delusions, especially of guilt, and hallucinations occur.

On the other hand, there are some severely depressed patients who do not accept their depression and utterly reject it. Technically, they should therefore not be considered psychotic. They are in this respect similar to the marginal schizophrenic who has at least partial insight into the pathological nature of his condition. However, both this type of severely depressed patient and schizophrenic patient can easily lose insight. If in the term psychosis we include the potential loss of insight, then they too can be called psychotic. If we do so, however, we step on unsafe ground. To obviate these difficulties, I suggest that we call a depression either mild or severe with the understanding that severe depression may be accepted by the patient as a way of living and therefore be syntonic, or unaccepted and therefore dystonic.

Our difficulties are not over. Many clinicians could correctly point out that many cases of depression cannot clearly be differentiated into mild or severe; rather, they reach an intermediate stage of intensity. Inasmuch as most cases could in their psychodynamic structure and clinical course resemble either the mild or the severe type of depression, I am inclined to classify these intermediate stages as moderate-to-mild depression and moderate-to-severe depression.

Are the age of the patient or particular contingencies in his life important to justify particular classifications? I mean, for instance, postpartum depression, adolescent depression, involutional depression, or senile depression, etc. They are justified only to the extent that they frequently have some specific clinical or psychodynamic features. It is important for the therapist to familiarize himself with them. However, the basic mechanisms are presumably the same as in other types of either mild or severe depression.

Table 3-1 demonstrates the classification adopted in this book. It also includes varieties which, although not necessary to distinguish for therapeutic reasons or for the understanding of their psychodynamics, have been recognized by several authors on account of their specific characteristics. They are reported here for the sake of clarification and to facilitate a common ground of understanding.

Before proceeding to a description of the clinical syndromes in Table 3-1, we shall briefly consider other classifications or attempts to classify depression.

Table 3-1

Classification of Depressions

Primary Depressions

Mild (dystonic)	a. Depressive Character or Personality
	b. Reactive Depression c. Depression with Anxiety
	d. Depression with ObsessiveCompulsive Symptoms
	e. Masked Depression
	f. Depersonalized Depression
Severe (syntonic)	a. Pure Depression

b. Depression in Manic-Depressive Psychosis

c. Depression in Schizo-Affective Psychosis

Varieties

1. Self-blaming
2. Claiming
3. Mixed
4. Simple
5. Acute
6. Agitated
7. Paranoid
8. With stupor

Related to the Cycle of Life	a. Childhood Depression
	b. Adolescent Depression
	c. Postpartum Depression
	d. Involutional Melancholia
	e. Senile Depression

Secondary Depressions

a. Depression with Neurological Disorders or Organic Psychoses

b. Depression with Endocrine Disorders c. Depression with Other Physical Illnesses

d. Drug-Induced Depression
e. Schizophrenic Depression

A classification based on genetic or biochemical mechanisms is not justified or possible at the present time. Frazier (1976) reminds us that

> A variety of hypotheses still exists about the role of chemical transmitter systems in the biology of depression, an area which has continued to be of interest to researchers. There has been a continuing debate between British and American psychiatrists regarding the relative role serotonin and norepinephrine play in the biology of depression.

In a very scholarly paper Akiskal and McKinney (1975) tried to integrate ten conceptual models of depression, but they failed to draw a classification based on chemistry or on theories which would explain the "leap from chemistry to behavior." They wrote that "biochemical statements that propose a causal relationship between a chemical event in the brain and a set of observable behaviors or subjective experiences present serious philosophical problems." They quote Smythies

(1973) in his assertion that attempts to explain mind only in terms of brain chemistry encounter irreducible and unsurmountable elements.

The Task Force on Nomenclature and Statistics of the American Psychiatric Association has proposed the following classification of mood disorders:

Unipolar manic disorder

296.01X	Single episode
296.02X	Recurrent

Unipolar depressive disorder

296.11X	Single episode
296.12X	Recurrent

Bipolar mood disorder

296.20X	Manic
296.30X	Depressed

296.40X	Mixed

Intermittent mood disorders

301.110	Intermittent depressive disorder
301.120	Intermittent hypomanic disorder
300.410	Demoralization disorder

Other mood disorders

300.420	Other depressive disorder
296.610	Other manic disorder
296.620	Other bipolar disorder

An "X" as the sixth digit indicates that the current condition is further specified as: 1 = mild; 2 = moderate; 3 = severe, but not psychotic; 4 = psychotic; 5 = in partial remission; 6 = in full remission.

I participated in the "Working Conference to

Critically Examine DSM-III in Midstream," which took place in St. Louis, Missouri on June 10-12, 1976. During the conference many participants objected to the classification proposed by the task force. The categories "intermittent mood disorders" seemed unclear and unnecessary to several participants who thought that these conditions are only mild forms of affective disorders. Many also objected to the proposed term "demoralization disorder" intended to designate neurotic depression. Maria Kovacs of the University of Pennsylvania School of Medicine stated, "The use of the word *demoralization* seems out of place. In a sense, every patient who recognizes his illness and comes for treatment is demoralized. According to the dictionary, demoralization means loss of morale, loss of psychological well-being because one has lost one's sense of purpose and confidence in the future, or loss of task-related attitudes expected and shared by one's group. By this definition, the concept is true of practically all psychiatric patients as well as numerous other people who might not exhibit long-term, chronic low self-esteem."

I also objected to the term "demoralization disorder," as well as to the term psychotic depression as it was described in the proposed nomenclature; that is, referring only to a condition that presents delusions and hallucinations. I repeated the same objections made earlier in this chapter.

I also stated that the term "mood disorders" seemed to me less appropriate than "affective disorders." First, the word mood as commonly used in English generally refers to the usual disposition of the personality and to the usual gamut of variations found within the limits of normality. The word affective has a deeper impact, more commensurate with the depth that affective disorders can reach. Secondly, it is one of the aims of DSM-III to preserve similarity with European nomenclatures. The word mood is very difficult to translate into foreign languages, especially those deriving from Latin. The French word *humeur* could not be used correctly. In several classifications the component *thymo,* from the Greek *thymos,* is used to mean affect. I suggested maintaining the term "affective disorders." I also pointed out that the use of the term unipolar to specify the disorders that have only depressive or manic episodes, although increasing in popularity, is incorrect and should be discouraged. Polarity means having or showing two contrary qualities, forms, or positions. The terms for two poles, like North Pole and South Pole, are called correlational terms; like husband and wife, one cannot exist without the other. If the earth were shaped like a pear, it would have one apex but not one pole. It is true that the term unipolar is used in electricity, but for something devised artificially. We would never say that a pear is unipolar. I suggested that the terms monophasic and biphasic be used instead of unipolar and bipolar.

Primary Depressions

Mild Depressions

Mild depressions can be classified into different types, but all or most of them share some characteristics which I shall describe here. Most conspicuous is the feeling of depression, except in those conditions called masked depressions and in syndromes of depersonalization.

Depression as a symptom is difficult to differentiate from the feeling of depression as a normal emotion, generally called sadness, which is part of the gamut of feelings of the average individual. Depression as a rule is experienced with greater intensity than sadness. It is an unpleasant feeling, difficult to overlook or shake off. It does not tend to fade away spontaneously except after a more or less prolonged period of time. As a matter of fact, the person who feels depressed often does not see how he will be able to get rid of his depressed feeling. Often it appears to him that he will remain depressed forever. Actually the opposite is true; in almost every case of mild depression the feeling sooner or later subsides or disappears completely. In many cases, however, it also recurs.

The second characteristic of mild depression is that the patient does not want to have such a despondent feeling; he rejects it, but does not know how to get rid of it. He recognizes that his symptom is unwarranted or exaggerated, and that it is a handicap and to some extent disruptive of the normal functions of life. In other words, he is aware of the dystonic nature of the symptom. The patient is generally correct in this regard: the depressive mood delays his spontaneous behavior and planned activities, requires an extra effort for concentration and work, keeps him distracted from what he would rather do or think, and leaves little room for other emotions. In some cases the patient is able to connect the depression with an event that almost everybody else also would consider unpleasant, but his reaction is nevertheless exaggerated. In Gutheil's words (1959) he is not only sad, but pessimistic. For Gutheil, pessimism is the added element that changes simple sadness into depression. We may add that this pessimism is often but not always accompanied by feelings of loneliness, unworthiness, and self-criticism.

Ideas that life is not worthwhile occur and suicidal projects present themselves, but not in an enduring fashion. Generally suicidal ideas are not carried out.

Psychosomatic and somatic symptoms accompany almost every case of depression. Appetite and eating habits change. In a large number of patients there is a noticeable but not excessive loss of weight. On the other hand, in a considerable number of patients there is a considerable increase in weight. The patient eats in an effort to assuage his depression.

Sleep dysfunction is also a frequent symptom. Many patients complain of insomnia;

yet they may sleep longer than usual, either because they do not want to face the day or because they really believe, at least at a manifest level, that their sleep requirements have increased. They claim that unless they sleep longer hours they feel fatigued, but fatigue remains a common symptom even if they do sleep longer than usual. Constipation is also a common complaint. Many mildly depressed patients complain of a decrease in sexual libido, and yet some of them indulge more than usual in sexual behavior in an attempt to find solace.

In addition to all or most of these characteristics, mild depressions have other traits that permit special classification. In some cases it is impossible to ascertain to what type the depression should be ascribed. The whole issue of whether such classification is warranted also is a matter of debate.

One of these varieties can be called depressive character (Bemporad, 1976) or depressive personality. In these cases, according to Bemporad, "depression appears to be a *constant* mode of feeling lurking in the background during everyday life." It is a conscious reaction to the loss of a state of well being. Contrary to some of the other character or personality disorders, the patient is dissatisfied with his condition and would like to change it. The unpleasant feeling often occurs after seemingly insignificant frustration. Bemporad reports that in the depressive character it is easy to find the primary triad of cognitive sets described by Beck (1967): a negative view of the world, the self, and the future.

The main feature of this variety of mild depression is its constant or almost constant character, so that the depressive mood becomes an important feature of the character. The patient is usually referred to as a depressed person. In some cases the patient does not describe himself as depressed, but as a person who is bored and has lost "la joie de vivre," or sees no possibility of joyful excitement in his life.

The variety of depression which we are going to describe now has received much more consideration in psychiatric literature—that is, reactive depression. This condition is characterized chiefly by the fact that it starts after the occurrence of an unpleasant happening in the life of the patient, or after an event which is considered by the patient to be adverse or unwelcome.

Bereavement, or loss through death of a person dear to the patient, is probably the most common precipitating factor of reactive depression. As we shall describe in greater detail in chapter 5, sadness due to mourning is a normal experience. Whereas the normal person sooner or later recovers from the experience of grief, however, the person who becomes depressed finds himself unable to shake off this unpleasant feeling. On the contrary, the anguish lingers and may become even more severe.

In my experience reactive depression connected with marital difficulties is very common. Also frequent is the depression over the end of a love relation, or over the loss of the loved person as an object of love. Loss of employment, disappointments at work, lack of promotion, financial difficulties, breaking up an important friendship, loss of status and prestige, and insults received are precipitating factors of reactive depression that can be easily understood even at a reality level.

The situation is more complex when the loss apparently does not justify the intensity of the depression; for instance, when the death of a bird, the loss of a handkerchief, or the inability to get tickets for a show provoke a depression. It seems easy to conclude in these cases that the precipitating event has a symbolic value, as we shall see in greater detail later in this book. In some cases of reactive depression other symptoms occur often, but not always: irritability, anger, an insatiable desire to get or obtain, and even a desire to alienate or manipulate others.

Another type of mild depression is "depression with anxiety." It consists of a clinical picture in which depression and anxiety occur concurrently. It is generally included under the group of depressions if the depressive mood is the prevailing one, although anxiety plays an important role in the total picture. In addition to being depressed, the patient is anxious, worried, expects something bad to happen, and is generally fearful of his own usual activities. In some instances he gives the impression of preferring to be depressed rather than anxious, and that the depression is an escape from anxiety. However, if the depression reaches great proportions, it may become more intolerable than the anxiety.

Another variety, more frequent than it would seem from cases reported in the literature, is the combination of depression and obsessive-compulsive symptoms. In addition to being depressed, the patient presents obsessions, compulsions, and rituals of the obsessive-compulsive kind. Contrary to what occurs in typical cases of obsessive-compulsive psychoneurosis, the obsessive and especially the compulsive symptoms are not very resistant. In some cases at least they are more easily overcome in obsessive-compulsive depression than in a typical obsessive-compulsive psychoneurosis.

Obsessive-compulsive depression is not uncommon in very religious persons who have learned to practice rituals in a compulsive way. Some of these cases are not mild and can be classified more properly as cases of severe depression in which obsessive-compulsive symptoms also appear.

The next two types of depression are characterized by the absence of depression as a feeling state of which the patient is aware. The first of these conditions is called masked depression. Doubts about the existence of such a clinical entity stem not only from different criteria of classification, but also from semantic and philosophical sources. In fact, can we talk of a feeling which is not felt? Can we talk of a felt experience which is not experienced? Freud too felt that an idea may become unconscious but an emotion by definition must always be felt.

In 1944 Kennedy reported that in many patients the symptomatology consists almost exclusively of somatic dysfunctions, which he called manic-depressive equivalents. Such terms as masked, hidden, or missed depression have appeared especially in the German literature. In 1937 Hempel published a paper on depression in which he characterized autonomic nervous disorders, and in 1949 Lemke wrote about depression of the vegetative system. Perhaps imitating the terminology used in reference to epilepsy, Ibor Lopes (1966) wrote about depressive equivalents and of *depressio sine depressione.*

According to Berner, Katschnig, and Poldinger (1973) most of the authors who use the expression masked depression mean "a depression in which the physical manifestations conceal the psychopathological symptomatology." Other people mean "a depression not recognized by a previous examiner who believed it to be a somatic disease." Still others call masked depression "any depression characterized by masked physical signs and symptoms." These are circular definitions. When we say that masked depression is a depression characterized by physical symptomatology, we offer only a tautologic statement deprived of any explanatory value. In fact we would have to demonstrate that the physical symptomatology is indeed a form of depression.

Geisler (1973) made a study of patients suffering from masked depression who were diagnosed as suspected of suffering from internal diseases such as angina pectoris, autonomic nervous dystonia, cardiovascular disorders, cholecystitis, colitis, diverticulitis, food allergy, neoplasm, and pernicious anemia. Thirty-six patients suffering from masked depression complained of sleep disorders, lack of appetite, abdominal symptoms, anxiety, cardiac symptoms, constipation, and so on. According to Geisler, the most frequent combination of symptoms consisted of complaints referring to organs, sleep disorders, poor appetite, and anxiety.

According to Braceland (1966) the six most frequent symptoms of masked depression are insomnia, tiredness, gastric and epigastric discomfort, anorexia, headache, and general abdominal pain. In many of these cases the differential diagnosis from hypochondriasis or psychosomatic conditions is difficult to make. In some cases the diagnosis reflects the classificatory habits of the therapist more than the nature of the condition.

In my opinion a common form of masked depression is the condition which is generally referred to as alcoholism. A considerable number of depressed people hide their depression by making immoderate use of alcohol, and therefore they are considered alcoholic. They often reveal their depression during the alcohol-free intervals. That they are fundamentally depressed also is revealed by the fact that most of them respond satisfactorily to antidepressants like imipramine.

An uncommon type of depression without depressive feeling is one which often assumes the characteristics of the syndrome of depersonalization. The person no longer feels like himself. Sensations are dull; perceptions are changed; reality may appear modified or transformed; a sense of distance and of space seems unreal. The person's voice or part of his body seems not to belong to him. The patient is depersonalized insofar as he has the feeling that he is not the same person and he cannot think, feel, act, or be motivated as he used to be. Up to this point the picture seems unrelated to depression, but the fact is that at times the patient does feel depressed. Another characteristic that suggests the depressive nature of this syndrome is the fact that some of these patients (but not all) respond well to electric shock treatment, at least for a temporary remission. They also improve with amphetamine and amphetamine derivatives. By no means is it implied here that all or even most patients suffering from depersonalization are depressed.

There is an additional remark to be made about both masked depression and depersonalization. It is more than doubtful that if they belong to the category of depression, they should be included under the group of mild rather than severe depressions. In some of these cases the symptomatology is quite marked and incapacitating.

Severe Depression

Severe depression as a clinical entity has been known since antiquity. Its features are generally very pronounced, easily recognizable, and much more easily definable than those of mild depression.

What seems to have remained unchanged from the time of Hippocrates to the late 1950s is a picture of an intense state of depression in which one can almost always recognize a profound and overwhelming theme of selfblame, hopelessness, and self-depreciation. Although cases with this classic picture are still very common, others—with a picture which I call claiming depression—occur with increasing frequency.

We shall review the various syndromes of severe depression with the understanding that the division into types and varieties is not very well established and in many cases still a matter of controversial debate.

Classic Form Of Severe Depression

Severe depression is characterized by the following triad of psychological symptoms: (1) a pervasive feeling of melancholia; (2) a disorder of thought processes, characterized by retardation and unusual content; and (3) psychomotor retardation. In addition there are accessory somatic dysfunctions.

The pervasive mood of depression at times has its onset quite acutely and dramatically, at other times slowly and insidiously. The patient generally has had previous attacks of depression which, because they were mild in intensity, passed unnoticed or were considered by the patient and his family as normal variations of mood. Even an attack that will later appear severe in intensity is misunderstood at first. An unpleasant event has occurred, such as the death of a close relative or a grief of any kind, and a mood of sadness is justified. However, when a certain period of time has elapsed and the unhappy feeling should have subsided, it seems instead to become more intense. The patient complains that he cannot think freely, feels unable to work, cannot eat, and sleeps only a few hours a night.

As the symptoms increase in intensity, the

patient himself may request to be taken to a physician. Often, however, the illness is advanced to such a degree that the patient no longer is able to make such a decision and he consults a physician at the initiative of family members. When the physician sees the patient, he is impressed by his unhappy, sad appearance. The patient looks older than his age, his forehead is wrinkled, and his face, although undergoing very little mimic play, reveals a despondent mood. In some cases the main fold of the upper eyelid at the edges of its inner third is contracted upward and a little backward (sign of Veraguth).

In most cases the examiner is led astray by the complaints of the patient, which consist of physical pain, a feeling of discomfort, digestive difficulties, lack of appetite, and insomnia. The physician may interpret these complaints as simple psychosomatic dysfunctions. They may persist and constitute a syndrome of severe masked depression. In the majority of cases, however, the mood of melancholia sooner or later becomes prominent and leads to an easy diagnosis.

The patient is often at a loss to describe the experience of melancholia. He says that his chest is heavy, his body is numb; he would like to sleep, but he cannot; he would like to immerse himself in activities, but he cannot; he would even like to cry, but he cannot. "The eyes have consumed all the tears." "Life is a torment." There is at the same time a desire to punish oneself by destroying oneself, which at the same time would end one's suffering. Suicidal ideas occur in about 75 percent of patients, and actual suicide attempts are made by at least 10 to 15 percent. Often the suicide attempt occurs when it is not expected, because the patient seems to have made some improvement and the depression is less pronounced. In a minority of suicide attempts, the suicidal idea was carefully concealed from the members of the family. The desire to end life applies only to the life of the patient himself, with one important exception to be kept in mind always: young mothers who undergo psychotic depression often plan to destroy not only themselves but their children, who presumably are considered by the patient to be an extension of herself. Newspaper reports about mothers who have killed themselves and their little children in most cases refer to patients suffering from unrecognized attacks of severe depression.

The other important symptom of depression concerns the content and type of thinking. As far as the content is concerned, the thoughts of the patient are characterized by gloomy, morbid ideas. In some cases, at the beginning of the attack, ideas occur that at first may not be recognized as part of the ensuing picture of psychotic depression. They may be phobic, obsessive, or obscene. They are followed by discouraging ideas which acquire more and more prominence. The patient feels that he will not be able to work, he will lose his money, something bad will happen to his family, somebody is going to get hurt, or the family is in extreme poverty. There is no great variety in the patient's thoughts. It is almost as if the patient purposely selects the thoughts that have an unpleasant content. *They are not thoughts as thoughts; they are chiefly carriers of mental pain.*

The distortion caused by the unpleasantness of the mood at times transforms these melancholic thoughts into almost delusional ideas or into definite delusions. They often represent distortions of the body image and hypochondriasis. The patient thinks he has cancer, tuberculosis, syphilis, and so on. His brain is melting, his bowels have been lost, his heart does not beat. Delusions of poverty are also common. Ideas of guilt, sin, and selfcondemnation are very pronounced, especially in serious cases. At times these self-accusatory ideas are so unrealistic that the name "delusion" seems appropriate for them. "It is all my fault;" "It is all my responsibility." In some cases the tendency to blame oneself reaches the absurd; the patient blames himself for being sick or for "succumbing to the illness." In some cases, he feels that he is not really sick but he acts as if he were sick. This impression is almost the opposite of what we find in some schizophrenics, in whom there is the idea that the world is a big stage, and what happens in the world is an act or a play. The depressed patient, on the contrary, feels that he is acting the part of the sick person. Incidentally, this idea occurs generally when the patient starts to recover from his depressed attack.

These delusional ideas cannot always be traced back to an exaggeration or distortion of mood. In cases that have a mixed paranoid and melancholic symptomatology, the delusions are more inappropriate and bizarre and are in no way distinguishable from those of paranoid patients.

In a small percentage of severely depressed patients there are obsessive-compulsive thoughts, similar to those occurring in obsessivecompulsive psychoneuroses or in mild depression with obsessive features. The pervasive mood of depression prevails, however, in the context of the complex symptomatology.

In the classical or traditional type of psychotic depression, the main theme is a selfblaming attitude. In severe cases the patient seems to transmit the following message: "Do not help me. I do not deserve to be helped. I deserve to die." Together with this peculiar content of thought, there is a retardation of thinking processes. The patient complains that he cannot concentrate; he cannot focus his attention. At first he can read, but without retaining what he reads. Writing is more difficult for him and composing a letter requires tremendous effort. If the patient is a student, he cannot study any longer. Thoughts seem to follow each other at a very slow pace. Speech is also slow. In a severe state of stupor the patient cannot talk at all.

Hallucinations in severe depression are described by many authors, especially in the old textbooks. According to the experience of many psychiatrists, however, they are much less common in severe depression than they used to be. This difference is not apparent, in the sense that patients who hallucinate are now diagnosed as schizophrenics. I have found that hallucinations do occur, although rarely, in some severely depressed patients. They have the following characteristics:

1. They are very rare in comparison to their occurrence in schizophrenia.

2. They do not have the distinct perceptual and auditory quality that they have in schizophrenia. The patients often cannot repeat what the voices say; they sound indistinct. The patients describe them as "as if rocks were falling," or as "bells which ring." Often they seem more like illusions than hallucinations, or as transformations of actual perceptions.

3. They can be related to the prevailing mood of the patient much more easily than in schizophrenia. Their secondary character—that is, secondary to the overall mood—is obvious. They are generally depressive and denigratory in

content, often commanding selfdestruction or injury.

4. More frequently than in schizophrenic patients, they occur at night, less frequently during the day. The depressed patient, who is in contact with external reality more than the schizophrenic, possibly needs the removal of diurnal stimuli in order to become aware of these inner phenomena.

Another important sign of the classic type of depression consists of retarded hypoactivity. The actions of the patient decrease in number, and even those which are carried out are very slow. Even the perceptions are retarded. Talking is reduced to a minimum, although a minority of patients retain the tendency to be loquacious. Working at the usual daily tasks of life is postponed or retarded. The patient avoids doing many things but continues to do what is essential. Women neglect their housework and their appearance. Every change seems to require a tremendous effort. Interpersonal relations are cut off. In some less pronounced cases, however, the opposite at first seems to occur. The patient, who is prone to accuse himself and extoll others, becomes more affectionate toward the members of his family and willing to do many things for them in an unselfish manner. However, when the disorder increases in intensity later, he becomes indifferent to everybody.

The physical symptoms that accompany classic depressive attacks are reduction in sleep, decrease in appetite, and considerable loss in weight. These symptoms do not seem to be due to a specific or direct physiological mechanism, but rather are related to or are a consequence of the depression. Many patients complain of dryness of the mouth, which is to be attributed to decreased secretion of the parotid glands (Strongin and Hinsie, 1938).

Other frequent symptoms are constipation, backache, amenorrhea, and dryness of the skin. There is a definite decrease in sexual desire, often to the point of complete impotence or frigidity. In many patients sugar is found in the urine during the attack. The basal metabolism tends to be slightly lower than normal.

The Claiming Type Of Depression

As we have already mentioned, since the late 1950s there has been a decline in the number of cases showing the classic type of depression, either as part of manic-depressive psychosis or as part of pure depression. Moreover, the cases that we do see seldom reach those severe degrees which used to be very common. Another type of depression is frequently observed now, whose symptomatology has the appearance of an appeal, a cry for help. The patient is anguished but wants people near him to become very aware of his condition. All his symptoms seem to imply the message, "Help me; pity me. It is in your power to relieve me. If I suffer, it is because you don't give me what I need." Even the suicidal attempt or prospect is an appeal of "Do not abandon me" or, "You have the power to prevent my death. I want you to know it." In other words, the symptomatology, although colored by an atmosphere of depression, is a gigantic claim. Now it is the gestalt of depression that looms in the foreground with the claim lurking behind; now it is the claim which looms, with the depression apparently receding. Poorly hidden also are feelings of hostility for people close to the patient, such as members of the family who do not give the patient as much as he would like. If anger is expressed, feelings of guilt and depression follow. Whereas the patient with the self-blaming type of depression generally wants to be left alone, the claiming type of patient is clinging, dependent, and demanding. Selfaccusation and guilt feelings play a secondary role or no role at all in this type of depression.

Whereas in the self-blaming type of depression there is a decrease of appetite and insomnia, in the claiming type the appetite is not necessarily diminished and quite often there is a need and ability to sleep longer than usual. In some cases the patient does not want to get up from bed and wishes to return to it several times during the day.

Other Clinical Varieties Of Depression

Some authors distinguish several varieties of severe depression: the simple, the acute, the paranoid, and the depressive stupor.

Simple depression is characterized by the moderate intensity of symptoms and may make the diagnosis of psychosis difficult. Delusions and hallucinations are absent. Although there is psychomotor retardation, the patient is able to take care of his basic vital needs. Suicidal ideas and attempts also occur in this type. In recent years cases of simple depression seem to have increased in number.

In *acute depression* the symptoms are much more pronounced. Self-accusation and ideas of sin and poverty are prominent. Some depressive ideas bordering on delusion are present. The loss of weight is very marked.

In *paranoid depression,* although the prominent feature remains the depressed mood, delusional ideas play an important role. The patient feels that he is watched, spied on, or threatened. Somebody wants to hurt him. Hypochondriacal delusions with pronounced distortion of the body image may occur. As in the case of hallucinations, these delusions seem secondary to the prevailing mood of the patient. They disappear easily when the mood changes. Hallucinations may also occur.

Depressive stupor is the most pronounced form of depression. Here there is more than psychomotor retardation: the movements are definitely inhibited or suppressed. The patients are so absorbed in their own pervasive feelings of depression that they cannot focus their attention on their surroundings. They do not seem to hear; they do not respond. They are mute, with the exception of some occasional utterances. Even mimic expressions are absent and the face seems mask-like, in a way reminiscent of the faces of some postencephalitic and Parkinsonian patients. Since the patients cannot focus on anything, they give the impression of being apathetic, whereas they are actually the prey of a deep, disturbing emotion. These patients cannot take care of themselves. Generally they lie in bed mute and have to be spoon-fed.

Unless they are successfully treated during the attack, physical health may suffer severely. Patients lose up to a hundred pounds in certain cases; they are constipated, and their circulation is enfeebled.

All the types of depression that we have so far described are also characterized by a lack of manic features or episodes during their course.

Depressive Phase Of Manic-Depressive Psychosis

All the clinical varieties of severe depression that we have described also appear as the depressive phase of manic-depressive psychosis.

In manic-depressive psychosis the classic type of depression is probably the most frequent. However, the claiming type, or mixed selfblaming and claiming type, also appears with typical or atypical symptomatology, as well as forms of simple depression, acute depression, paranoid depression, and depressive stupor.

What chiefly characterizes the depression occurring in manic-depressive psychosis is that it is followed regularly or occasionally by manic episodes. Inasmuch as the depressive picture is not dissimilar to the ones so far described, this section will be devoted to examination of the manic episode. The manic attack is not an attack of depression. Nevertheless we shall describe it here because it is a frequent component of a syndrome in which primary severe depression is an important part.

In the manic attack, as in an attack of severe depression, the symptomatology is characterized by: (1) a change in mood, which is one of elation (2) a disorder of thought processes, characterized by flight of ideas and happy content; and (3) an increased motility. Accessory body changes also occur.

It is difficult in many instances to determine the beginning of the episode. The patient is often in a lively mood. He strikes the observer as being an extrovert, active individual who likes to talk a great deal and do many things. At the time of the attack, however, the over joyousness of the patient seems out of proportion and occasionally inappropriate; for instance, when he easily dismisses things which should make him sad and continues to be in his happy mood. The patient appears exuberant very sociable, and at times even succeeds in transmitting his happiness to the surrounding persons. This mood, however, is not constant or solid. We are not referring here to the alternations with depression, but to the fact that this euphoric mood may easily change into one of irritation or even rage and anger, especially when the patient becomes aware that the environment does not respond to his enthusiasm or does not react in accordance with the exalted opinion that he has of himself.

The thinking disorder is prominent and reveals itself in verbal productions. The patient talks very fast and cannot concentrate on any subject for more than a few seconds. Any marginal idea is expressed; any secondary, distracting stimulus affects the patient. The thoughts expressed are not disconnected but maintain some apparent ties. We can always determine that the ideas are connected by the elementary laws of association, but the talk as a whole is verbose, circumstantial, and not directed toward any goal or toward the logical demonstration of any point which is discussed. The ensemble of these thought and language alterations is called "flight of ideas."

Actually this type of verbal behavior has a goal—that of maintaining this superficial effervescent euphoria and escaping from intruding thoughts which may bring about depression. In less pronounced cases the patient realizes that he has unduly allowed details to interfere with the original goal of his conversation, and he tries to go back to it but again gets lost in many details.

In this incessant logorrhea, the patient makes jokes. The propensity toward associations leads to repeated clang associations which the patient uses to make jokes, puns, and so on (Arieti, 1950). In rare cases the lack of thought inhibition facilitates a certain artistic propensity which does not, however, lead to achievement because of the lack of concentration.

Lorenz and Cobb (1952) and Lorenz (1953), who made an accurate study of speech in manic patients, reported that in manic speech there is a quantitative change in the use of certain speech elements, namely: (1) a relative increase in the use of pronouns and verbs; (2) a relative decrease in the use of adjectives and prepositions; and (3) a high verb-adjective quotient (that is, the proportion of adjectives is decreased). These authors found no gross disorganization at the level of structural elements, and they postulated that the defect in manic speech occurs at higher integrative levels of language formulation. They concluded that, "If the assumption of a correlation between emotional states and verb-adjective quotient is correct, the manic patient's speech gives objective evidence of a heightened degree of anxiety."

The rapid association ability that the manic possesses enables him to grasp immediately some aspects of the environment which otherwise would pass unnoticed. The patient is in the paradoxical situation in which his ability to observe and grasp environmental stimuli has increased, but he cannot make use of it because of his distractibility.

The patient's thought content often reveals an exalted opinion of himself. The patient may boast that he is very rich, a great lover, a famous actor, a prominent businessman. These statements receive flimsy support. When asked to prove them, the patient attempts to do so but soon is lost in a web of unnecessary details. He may become excitable if he is reminded of the goal of the conversation. Disturbances of the sensorium are generally of minimal intensity and are caused by the exalted mood or distractibility, not by intellectual impairment.

Motor activity is increased. Manic patients are always on the go, in a state that ranges from mild motor excitement to incessant and wild activity. They talk, sing, dance, tease, destroy, move objects. In severe states these actions or movements remain unfinished and purposeless. In spite of their constant activity, manic patients do not feel tired and have tremendous endurance.

Accessory somatic symptoms consist of loss of weight which is generally not as pronounced as in depression, decrease in appetite, and constipation. Insomnia is marked. The blood pressure is generally lowered. Menses are irregular. Sexual functions, although apparently increased in hypomanic states, are generally decreased or disturbed in various ways in manic conditions.

Manic Varieties. As with depression, many forms of manic states have been described by early authors. A brief description of them follows.

In *hypomania* the symptoms are not of a marked intensity. As mentioned before, it is difficult at times to say whether the patient is showing his usual extrovert personality or the beginning of an illness. He seems full of pep and in good humor. He wants to do many things. His verbal abilities are accentuated. Although he has always had a talent for foreign languages, he now speaks many of them without hesitation, unconcerned with the mistakes he makes. Some of these patients increase their activities to such an exaggerated degree that they show very poor judgment. They are actually compelled by their inner excitability and by their exalted mood. They may walk for miles and miles. Generally they have a goal (for instance, to reach the next village), but not a necessary one. They may send out hundreds of unnecessary letters or greeting cards and make a large number of lengthy telephone calls. They often go on spending sprees, with disastrous economic consequences. Their sexual activity is increased, and lack of control may bring about unpleasant results. Illegitimate pregnancies in hypomanic women and venereal diseases in hypomanic men and women are relatively common.

The excitability, richness of movements, and euphoric mood give a bizarre flavor to the manic's behavior. A female patient, in order to show a sore to a physician, completely undressed in front of him. Occasionally even thefts and fraudulent acts are committed. The patient retains the ability to rationalize his actions, at times to such an extent that the layman is confused and believes in the patient's sanity.

In *acute mania* the symptoms are much more pronounced. They may accelerate gradually, from a previously hypomanic state, or rapidly, from a normal condition. The patient is in such a state of extreme restlessness that his behavior may be very disturbing and difficult to control. He may disrupt theatrical audiences, sing or scream in the street, or ring bells. If an attempt is made to control him, he may become belligerent. The mood is one of such exaltation that spontaneous thoughts of self aggrandizement are accepted immediately.

A subtype which Kraepelin differentiated from acute mania is delusional mania, characterized by an abundance of grandiose delusional ideas reminiscent of those found in the expansive type of general paresis.

Delirious mania represents an extreme stage of excitement. The patient is incoherent, disoriented, restless, and agitated. He may easily injure himself and others in his aimless activity. Restraint, chemical or physical, is an absolute necessity to avoid exhaustion which may lead to death. Hallucinations and delusions are frequent.

In addition to the types just mentioned, Kraepelin has described *mixed states* which are characterized by a combination of manic and depressive symptoms. He distinguishes the following six principal types: (1) manic stupor; (2) agitated depression; (3) unproductive mania; (4) depressive mania; (5) depression with flight of ideas; and (6) akinetic mania.

The names given to these types indicate the

combination of chief symptoms for each. Of the six types, perhaps the most common is agitated depression. In this condition a motor restlessness, typical of a manic excitement, is superimposed on a markedly depressive symptomatology.

Although the types of manic-depressive psychosis have been described as if they were separate entities, all the types are related, as Kraepelin saw when he first formulated the large nosological concept of manic-depressive psychosis.

The melancholic and the manic attack, which at first seem so different, have an intrinsic similarity; the same mental functions are altered, although the alterations are in a certain way opposite. Whereas in depression the mood is one of melancholia, in the manic attack it is one of elation; whereas in depression the thought processes and motor activity are retarded, in the manic attack a flight of ideas and increased motility are found.

One of the main characteristics of manicdepressive psychosis is the recurrence of the attacks, which has conferred to the disorder the designation, often used in Europe, of intermittent psychosis.

The attack may occur in different successions, which old books of psychiatry described at great length and with many illustrations that represented the manic attack as a positive wave and the depression as a negative wave. A sequence of a depressed phase followed by a manic phase is the typical pattern of circular psychosis. We may observe, however, that the attacks of depression far outnumber those of mania. Some patients may undergo a conspicuous number of depressions without ever having a manic phase.

There seems to be no relation between the duration of the attack and of normal intervals. At times, short attacks recur several times in short succession, but occasionally the series is interrupted by a long normal interval. I have seen several cases in which an attack of depression in the patient's early twenties was not followed by a second one until the patient had reached his middle sixties or even seventies. Kraepelin illustrated that many attacks of depression occurring later in life, which many authors consider as a subtype of senile psychosis, must instead be considered to be late occurrences or relapses of manic-depressive psychosis.

According to Pollock et al. (1939) 58.1 percent of patients have only one attack, 26.1 percent have two attacks, 9.3 have three attacks, and 6.5 percent have more than three attacks. Occasionally, one finds a patient who has had 25 or even more attacks.

The age at which the first attack occurs varies. It may even happen in childhood in rare cases. By far the largest number of first attacks occur between the ages of twenty and thirty-five. Manic attacks are slightly more frequent between the ages of twenty and forty. After forty, their ratio to depressive attacks decreases further. Women are more susceptible to this psychosis than men. (About 70 percent of patients are women.)

The illness generally results in recovery as far as the individual attack is concerned. Repeated attacks usually cause very little intellectual impairment. Death, however, may occur in two instances: suicide in depression, and exhaustion or cardiac insufficiency in cases of delirious mania. Another situation which we shall discuss later is the change of the manicdepressive symptomatology into a schizophrenic one, either shortly after the onset of the illness or even after many years of hospitalization.[7]

Prognostic criteria as to the future course of the condition are very difficult when the patient is examined only from the point of view of manifest symptomatology. Contrary to what happens in schizophrenia, the manifest symptomatology of manic-depressive psychosis will rarely permit prediction as to whether the patient will have only the present attack, a few, or many in his lifetime. The prognosis is almost always good as to the individual attack, but it is uncertain as to the possibility of recurrence. Rennie (1942) in an accurate statistical study found that the prognosis is worse when attacks occur after the age of forty. He found that 70 percent of all patients had a second attack; 63.5 percent a third; and 45 percent a fourth. The more frequent the attacks, the worse the prognosis is.

Involutional Melancholia

A common type of depression occurs during

the climacterium (menopause), or shortly before or after, and is generally called involutional melancholia. This diagnosis was made more frequently in the past, before the advent of electric shock treatment, drug therapy, or psychotherapy on a large scale. Patients were admitted to psychiatric hospitals where at times they remained for very long periods of time, in some cases even for the rest of their lives. The majority of patients remained sick from one to five years. I myself while working at Pilgrim State Hospital saw many patients so diagnosed who had remained in the hospital for even more than ten years. The advent of electric shock treatment dramatically changed the picture and permitted the complete loss of symptomatology which had persisted for so long. All the mentioned types of treatment have drastically changed the course of the illness and permit a much more favorable prognosis.

Involutional melancholia is a syndrome characterized by severe depression which generally occurs for the first time during the socalled involutional age—between the ages of forty to fifty-eight in women, and fifty to sixtyfive in men. It is much more common in women.

The onset may be gradual and be manifested by anxiety, apprehension, hypochondriasis, and in some cases by quasiparanoid attitudes toward acquaintances, relatives, friends, co-workers, and so forth. Irritability and pessimism predominate at first, together with an excessive preoccupation with bodily functions and a fear of illnesses. Restlessness and frank motor agitation subsequently become the main feature in most cases. Psychomotor retardation, typical of other severe types of depression, is absent in many cases or not very pronounced. However, the patient is definitely less active than before the onset of the illness. The lack of purposeful activity at times contrasts with the motor restlessness. Female patients often are prompt to attribute their symptoms to menopause and to minimize psychological factors of any sort. In some cases that run a very acute and serious course, the examiner feels he is dealing with a person who considers his/her life already coming to an end. The remaining years are seen as a prolonged agony which it would be better to terminate with a self-imposed coup de grace.

In the past the most pronounced forms of depression were seen in involutional melancholia even more than in the depressive phase of manic-depressive psychosis or in other types of severe depression. Prior to the introduction of three types of treatment—electric shock treatment, drug therapy, and psychotherapy—the current belief of the medical staff in psychiatric hospitals was that only "about one-third of hospitalized cases lived through their psychosis to survive" (Bigelow, 1959). We must remember that these were hospitalized cases, and that this evaluation did not include milder cases which were never hospitalized. Today the prognosis is quite different. If suicide is avoided, recovery or very marked improvement occurs in 100 percent of cases.

In early studies of this condition, the prepsychotic personality of the involutional patient was described as being characterized by rigid adherence to the ethical code, narrow range of interests, meticulousness, stubbornness, and poor sexual adjustment (Titley, 1936). Others stressed obsessional, sadomasochistic, introverted personalities (Palmer and Sherman, 1938). Rosenthal (1968, 1974), who has made recent studies of involutional melancholia, does not give much credit to the findings of Palmer and Sherman and of Titley. He states that "one is hard-pressed to find any recent studies that confirm these findings with more sophisticated statistical techniques."

In addition, all the studies that relate involutional depression to the physical changes of the menopause or to other endocrine functions have led to no conclusive results.

Senile Depression

Senile depression must be distinguished from a depression which occurs in a predominantly organic condition, such as senile psychosis or cerebral arteriosclerosis.

Senile depression is a rather frequent form of generally moderate to severe depression, which is distinguished from the other types of severe depression because it occurs in old age in individuals who have not suffered from depression previously. It is characterized at first by psychosomatic and hypochondriacal preoccupations, followed by an overpowering feeling of depression, guilt, self-deprivation, inhibition of activity, retardation, and marked decrease in interest. At least two-thirds of the patients are women.

Some cases are relatively benign and are often diagnosed as cases of reactive depression because they occur after an unpleasant event has taken place. The most severe cases do not seem to be reactive to any specific event; rather, they seem to represent the unfavorable outcome of an entire life.

In a study reported by Charatan (1975) 52 percent of the patients who had been seen in a geriatric psychiatric outpatient clinic were diagnosed as suffering from an affective disorder —primarily psychotic depression.

In a considerable number of patients who are approaching old age, but who cannot yet really be called old—from their late fifties to middle sixties—the depression seems to be predominantly precipitated by sexual dysfunction or at least sexual preoccupations. Male patients complain that they have difficulty in erecting or that they lose the erection rapidly, ejaculate without strength or momentum, or without enough semen. Women complain of dyspareunia, complete frigidity, or even of total sexual disgust. In a minority of cases in both sexes there is also compulsive masturbation or even promiscuity in an attempt to overcome the depression. In many other cases, especially for widowers, loneliness is a much more frequent complaint than sexual dysfunction.

Postpartum Depression

All kinds of affective conditions may occur after childbirth, from the so-called postpartum blues to mania and psychotic depression. Inasmuch as I consider childbirth to be a precipitating event of great psychological significance although not physically related to the depression, postpartum depression is here included among the primary depressions.

The manifest symptomatology of postpartum depression is fundamentally not different from that of other severe depressions. In most cases there is a gradual increase of depressive characteristics. In some cases the condition is recognized several weeks after childbirth and only when a full-blown depression is present.

Frequent symptoms are insomnia, restlessness, hypoactivity, and disinterest or neglect of the child. In some cases there are also phobic and obsessive symptoms, which are quite distressing: the patient is afraid of harming or even killing the child. In less severe cases the patient is afraid that she will not be able to take care of her child. She considers herself a bad or unworthy mother. She either pities the child very much or is completely indifferent to him and considers him an intruder in her life. In still other cases the anxiety about not being able to be a good mother prevails over the feeling of depression.

In the most severe cases a deep depression, often accompanied by guilt and a total feeling of hopelessness, obliterates all other sensations.

Some postpartum depressions recover quite quickly, but most of them are of longer duration than other depressions and of severe intensity, irrespective of whether the depression is monophasic or part of a biphasic manicdepressive psychosis that has been precipitated by childbirth.

A very important distinction must be made in cases of postpartum depression in regard to the safety of the baby. If the patient in an obsessive or phobic way is afraid of hurting or even killing her child, the danger is minimal or practically nonexistent. The patient has to be reassured and told that she is suffering from a fear, not from a determination to do anything harmful. On the other hand, if the patient has no obsessive-compulsive or phobic symptoms, is very depressed, and expresses or nourishes suicidal ideas, the risk is great not only for her but also for the baby. What we mentioned before — that depressed women who commit suicide often include their children in the suicidal act and kill them too—applies especially in postpartum depressions. Twin babies are killed by depressed mothers just as easily as single children. The greatest surveillance is necessary.

Since all types of psychiatric conditions can occur after childbirth, the diagnosis may be difficult in atypical cases. The first diagnostic task consists in ascertaining whether the condition is a postpartum delirium, generally organic in nature, or any other psychiatric condition less frequently associated with organic factors. Delirium, which is characterized generally by confusion, extreme excitement, incoherent or irrelevant thinking, and a rather acute course, has become much less frequent in the last few decades probably because of improved obstetrical care and less probability of toxic conditions during pregnancy. The presence of schizophrenic symptoms such as delusions, hallucinations, or ideas of reference may lead easily to the diagnosis of schizophrenia.

However, many authors differ in their reports of the incidence of schizophrenic and affective psychoses after childbirth. According to Davidson (1936), schizophrenic and manic depressive psychoses each constituted 30 percent of postpartum psychiatric disorders. For Boyd (1942), manic-depressive psychosis constituted 40 percent, schizophrenia 20 percent, and delirium 28.5 percent. Strecker and Ebaugh (1926) reported 34 percent delirium, 36 percent manic-depressive, and 20 percent schizophrenic. Protheroe (1969) in England reported almost twice as many cases of affective psychosis as of schizophrenic psychosis. In a review article, Herzog and Detre (1976) state that the discrepancy between English and American statistics may be due to the fact that American clinicians have tended to underdiagnose the incidence of affective disorders and overdiagnose schizophrenia. In my opinion, an additional confusion results from the inability to make a differential diagnosis between manic-depressive psychosis and a depression which is not related to manicdepressive psychosis.

It is a common belief that postpartum conditions are less common today, and as a matter of fact there are many fewer reports about these conditions in the current psychiatric literature than in the literature of a few decades ago. However, according to my clinical experience, this belief is not correct: perhaps postpartum deliriums and full-fledged psychoses are less common because prenatal care and medical assistance during labor and puerperium have improved. Although I have not been able to develop adequate statistics, my bona fide impression is that less pronounced postpartum conditions are common, and that schizophrenic and affective psychoses are not at all rare.

Suicide

A relatively frequent outcome of severe depression is suicide, which we have already considered in relation to the self-blaming type of depression. We shall consider it here as part of the manifest symptomatology of every severe depression. The psychodynamics of suicide will be studied in chapters 6 and 8.

The occurrence of suicide in all types of severe depression is estimated variously. Rennie (1942) gave a conservative estimate of 5 percent in patients suffering from severe depression. According to Weiss (1974) more than 20,000 suicides are recorded each year in the United States, but Dublin (1963) has estimated that the correct number is 25,000, and Choron (1972) that it is 30,000. If we add to this number the attempted suicides whose exact number cannot be evaluated, we can conclude that the problem is of vast proportions indeed.

Although people who attempt successfully or unsuccessfully to commit suicide are by no means all depressed persons, the depressed constitute by far the largest group. Feelings of helplessness, hopelessness, failure, and willingness to face death as the only way out are prominent in people who make suicidal attempts. Unfavorable prognostic signs are the seriousness of the depression, a history of previous attempts, the seriousness of intention, advanced age, and old age. The risk increases when the patient is alone and feels that nobody will oppose his plans, and when his depression has decreased in intensity to such a point that he does not feel slowed down in his motor actions or at least in his physical ability to carry out the suicide attempt. Opportunities that facilitate the attempt are also dangerous, like living on a high floor, having a large amount of sleeping pills, the possibility of drowning oneself, or the availability of guns and ropes.

Secondary Depression

Depression With Neurological Or Brain Disease

Depressions accompanying neurological disease are relatively common. Perhaps the most common is the depression occurring in various types of epilepsy. It is less common in epileptics suffering from grand mals, perhaps because the fits have antidepressant effects, like the convulsions produced by ECT. Depression is relatively common in epileptics suffering from petit mals or psychomotor equivalents, or in patients whose electroencephalograms reveal diencephalic dysfunction or discharges from the temporal lobes.

The risk of suicide in depressed epileptics is very high because the patient has to contend not only with the depression but with the impulsive urges of the epileptic personality. Whether the depression occurring in epileptics is precipitated by the discomfort of the illness itself, or is an epileptic equivalent, or is just a depression that happens to occur in an epileptic person is difficult to determine in the majority of cases. These patients constitute serious therapeutic challenges.

In patients suffering from Huntington's chorea, depressions with suicidal attempts are quite common, especially for female patients (Whittier, 1975). Depression often is seen in postencephalitics. According to Brill (1975) these patients are characteristic for their whining voice, clinging manner, and dependent and complaining attitude. Hypochondriacal symptoms, self-accusations, and delusions of guilt are also common. Neal (1942) found that the most frequent clinical picture was similar to that described by Brill. However, in his review of 201 cases he found that pathological depression was reported nine times, psychotic depression eight times, and hypomania eight times.

Mild to moderate depression and even severe depression is common in patients suffering from Parkinson's disease. This finding, and the observation that depression often follows the use of drugs which affect the basal ganglia, have led to interesting hypotheses about the anatomical and biochemical nature of depression.

Many other chronic neurological diseases (muscular dystrophies, cerebellar atrophies) are accompanied by depression. In most cases the main therapeutic task is one of rehabilitation or adjustment to the condition. In many cases of multiple sclerosis, there is no depression in spite of the crippling features of the disease. On the contrary, the patient seems apathetic or nonchalant to his condition. Depression occurs also in mental defectives who are not so defective as to disregard their condition.

Depressed episodes occur in senile dementia and also in psychoses with cerebral arteriosclerosis. These depressive episodes do not last long and are generally not prominent in the general clinical picture. The patient feels mistreated, cries over alleged thefts of which he is a victim, and is confused.

Depression With Endocrine And Other Chronic Diseases

The thyroid is the endocrine gland more frequently involved in depressions that accompany endocrine disorders.

Hypothyroidism of any kind can lead to depression, especially when myxedema occurs. Hyperthyroidism (whether or not it reaches the clinical level of Graves' disease) is often complicated by depression. The patient's despondent mood is often accompanied or alternated by a mood of irritability and capriciousness.

I also have seen cases of depression in hyperparathyroidism and severe diabetes. Depression also occurs after coronary disease, although not so frequently as states of anxiety.

Many diseases, especially those running a chronic course, can be accompanied by depression. In all these cases it is difficult to determine whether the physical illness is etiologically related to depression or whether depression is merely a precipitating factor, that is, merely the patient's psychological response to the unpleasantness caused by his physical illness.

Drug-Induced Depression

The following drugs induce a depressive mood in some patients: steroids, chlorpromazine (Thorazine®), the butyrophenones like haloperidol (Haldol®), and especially the rauwolfia derivatives, like reserpine (Serpasil®). The depression is generally not severe and disappears with discontinuance of the drug.

Depression Occurring In The Course Of Schizophrenia

Depression may occur in the course of schizophrenia. It must be distinguished from schizo-affective psychosis, a condition in which a mixture of schizophrenic and manic-depressive symptoms takes place from the onset of the illness. Many psychiatrists, including myself, do not as a rule consider the occurrence of depression in the course of schizophrenia in negative terms but, on the contrary, as a sign of growth and good prognosis, especially if it occurs after the patient has started to respond favorably to treatment and the schizophrenic symptoms have disappeared or diminished in intensity.

Differential Diagnosis

The diagnosis is made in two steps. The first step consists of determining whether the patient is really suffering from a depression or from a syndrome simulating a depression. A person who seems depressed is not necessarily depressed in the clinical sense.

He may be experiencing normal sadness (see chapter 5). He may also be depressed and suffering from many psychiatric disorders, not necessarily just from a clinical form of depression. Depression, like anxiety, is found as a concomitant symptom in most psychiatric conditions. However, we are justified in calling a syndrome depression when the depressive mood constitutes the main characteristic, irrespective of whether this mood belongs to a primary or secondary form of depression.

Once we have ascertained that the patient is suffering from a real depression (and not from another syndrome), we proceed to the second step: What kind of depression is he suffering from?

An elderly person has lost a considerable amount of weight, looks depressed, and complains that he may have cancer. He may be mistaken for a person suffering from severe depression when he indeed has some kind of malignancy. If he also has depression, it may be precipitated by his appraisal of his poor physical condition. An accurate physical examination will determine the situation. In psychiatric practice, however, the opposite occurrence is more common: an elderly patient has lost weight, has many hypochondriacal complaints including a fear of cancer, and is depressed. Negative physical findings, psychomotor retardation, insomnia, and a despondent mood generally will determine that he is suffering from depression.

Some post-encephalitic patients and some parkinsonian patients are mistaken for depressed, even when their condition is not complicated by depression. The confusion is caused by the fact that patients with extrapyramidal syndromes have symptoms and signs which are reminiscent of characteristics found in depressed patients. These symptoms include loss of accessory movements, mask-like expression on the face, slow gait, posture with stooped body and flexed head, and general psychomotor retardation. Neurological examination and the medical history of the patient will lead to the correct diagnosis.

The complete or almost complete

immobility of the patient and a minimal response to external stimuli may make difficult a differential diagnosis between depressive stupor and catatonic stupor. Generally a history of depression leads to the diagnosis of depression, but not always; many catatonics have experienced some episodes of mild or severe depression before the catatonic attack. Often other concomitant symptoms such as negativism, the assumption of bizarre postures, the swelling of legs from standing, the closing of eyes, and the almost absolute absence of emotion lead to the diagnosis of catatonic stupor.

The diagnosis of schizophrenia is also to be ruled out in some cases of manic-depressive psychosis that resemble the schizophrenic syndrome, especially if manic phases occur. During the manic attack the patient's behavior may appear bizarre and there may be disorganization of thought processes. However, both behavior and thought processes are much more altered in schizophrenia. If hallucinations occur in manic-depressive psychosis, they have the differential characteristics mentioned previously; if paranoid ideation is present, it is only minimal. The total picture, including personality type which is cyclothymic in the case of manic-depressive psychosis, will lead to an easy diagnosis except for those cases that are usually placed in the schizo-affective category.

Once we have determined that we are dealing with a depression, we must proceed to the second step and ascertain the specific type of depression. The presence of another illness (for example, epilepsy or myxedema) will lead easily to the diagnosis of secondary depression. In the majority of cases it is not difficult to determine whether a particular case is one of mild (neurotic) or severe (psychotic) depression.

According to the *Diagnostic and Statistical Manual of Mental Disorders* of the American Psychiatric Association (DSM-n) (Committee on Nomenclature, 1968), the differentiation between psychotic depression and depressive neurosis "depends on whether the reaction impairs reality testing or functional adequacy enough to be considered a psychosis."

The reality testing in this case concerns the mood of depression. Does the patient consider his depression justified; does he want to maintain it; does it drastically transform his appreciation of life? If the answers is yes, the diagnosis is bound to be one of severe depression (psychotic depression) or manicdepressive psychosis. A history of manic attacks, or at least of a cyclothymic personality, will lead to the diagnosis of manic-depressive psychosis. In mild depression we can recognize the following differential characteristics which rule out a severe depression. (1) The depression is not so intense as to affect the total personality of the patient.

The patient wants to get rid of the depression. (3) Suicidal ideas are not a predominant feature. (4) The patient responds, although to a moderate degree, to cheerful aspects of the environment and to attempts to comfort him. (5) The psychosomatic symptoms are different inasmuch as (a) The loss of appetite is not excessive. In some cases there is increased appetite, (b) As a rule there is no premorbid anxiety, (c) The insomnia is relatively mild. In some cases there is an increased need to sleep, (d) There is no dryness of the mouth, (e) The constipation is less marked, (f) The skin is not dry. (g) There is no hypomenorrhea or amenorrhea.

Notes

[7] There are many psychiatrists who would deny such a statement.
 They feel that if a manic-depressive seems later to become schizophrenic, it is because the right diagnosis (schizophrenia) was not made. A considerable number of psychiatrists would call such a patient schizo-affective. Most psychiatrists, however, limit the diagnosis of schizoaffective psychoses to patients who present a mixed symptomatology from the beginning of the illness.

[4]

MANIFEST SYMPTOMATOLOGY OF DEPRESSION IN CHILDREN AND ADOLESCENTS

Jules Bemporad

The conceptual status of depression in childhood is somewhat ambiguous. Some authors (Rochlin, 1959; Beres, 1966) doubt that depression is possible in children on theoretical grounds. For example, these authors believe that prior to the establishment of the superego, self-directed aggression (which for them is the *sine qua non* of depression) is not possible and therefore young children cannot become truly depressed. Others believe that children cannot sustain a prolonged dysphoric mood and will vigorously find ways of escaping from depression. From a cognitive point of view, the lack of future orientation and

the "here and now" orientation make the possibility of self-perpetuating, clinical

depression in children less than likely. These questions are pursued further in chapter 8. This chapter will limit itself to a phenomenological description of childhood and adolescent syndromes which have been labeled as similar to the depressive disorders seen in adults.

Depressionlike States of Infancy

In 1946 Rene Spitz published a pioneering paper on the reaction of infants to maternal separation, thus opening up an avenue of productive research that continues today. He described children who had formed a normal attachment to their mothers and who subsequently were separated from their mothers at six months of age. Spitz reported that such infants responded with weepy, complaining behavior that eventually gave way to withdrawal and lethargy. In this latter condition the infants would lie in their cots with their faces averted, ignoring their surroundings. If approached by strangers, the infants would begin crying and screaming. If an infant was not reunited with his mother, he gradually developed a syndrome that Spitz called "anaclitic depression" which was characterized by weight loss, insomnia, a lack of response to people, and a frozen expression with a far-away gaze. Spitz reported that if the mother and infant were reunited after three to five months, the syndrome was reversible. If the separation continued after this amount of time, however, the infant's condition consolidated and became irreversible. Later these children showed arrests in various areas of development as well as a greater susceptibility to disease.

Spitz cautioned that while the symptoms manifested by these infants are similar to adult depressions, this form of depression differs from adult episodes in that it lacks the major factor of the adult disorder, the formation of a cruel superego. Spitz did speculate, however, that the child turns his aggression on himself because he lacks an external maternal object who can both absorb his aggressive drives and elicit a strong libidinal response to neutralize the aggressive instinctual forces. A decade later Engel and Reichsman (1956) described a similar symptom picture in a socially deprived infant girl, Monica, who also had a gastric fistula. These authors were not impressed by a presence of a retroflexed anger; rather, they postulated the presence of a basic "depression-withdrawal reaction" as the infant's attempt to shut out an unpleasant environment.

These reports stimulated much thinking and research regarding the appearance of infantile depressionlike episodes subsequent to maternal separation. One of the most prolific writers on this topic is Bowlby who has carefully studied and documented the process of infantile attachment to and separation from the mother figure. Bowlby (1958) has attempted to reformulate the infant's attachment to its mother along ethological concepts such as innate responses to certain releasing stimuli. In this manner the mother elicits instinctual attachment behavior in the infant, and the infant in turn sets off innate attachment behavior in the mother. The novelty in Bowlby's approach is that he views emotional attachment as independent of oral satisfaction, and he documents the specific behaviors that play a part in the attachment process.

In addition, Bowlby has documented the steps that follow abnormal separation from the mother (1960/;), and it is in this field that his work may have relevance for the study of infant depression. Bowlby proposes three stages in the separation process. First, in the stage of protest the infant is very upset and tries to reinitiate contact with the mother by crying, screaming, and thrashing about. The stage of despair follows quickly, during which the infant still seems to hope to be reunited with its mother. At this time, however, the crying is quieter and less constant. The infant gradually becomes silent, decreases its movements, and appears acutely depressed. In the final stage of defense or detachment, the child seems to have overcome his loss and will respond to other adults. He becomes cheerful and sociable once again. However, at this point the infant no longer selects out the mother and may in fact ignore her if she returns.

It would appear that Bowlby is describing the same behavior previously reported by Spitz and by Engel and Reichsman. However, Bowlby makes some crucial interpretations that differ from the previous researchers. He does not consider this behavior to represent an infantile prototype of depression, but rather to demonstrate a universal form of mourning secondary to separation. He describes a more benign prognosis than Spitz; he notes that children overcome the traumatic separation without long-range developmental retardation. In fact Bowlby speculates that such children, if they are subjected to recurrent separation, form progressively less attachment to mother figures and eventually become nonfeeling, non-empathic psychopaths—rather than depressed adults. As early as 1937 David Levy described just such an individual in the case of an eight-year-old girl who had been in a succession of foster homes and could not form a loving relationship with her adopted parents. Levy described this girl as exhibiting a lack of emotional reactiveness together with an "affect hunger," or a need to be given to by others. Since Levy's initial description other similar cases have been reported, and Bowlby has supplied these clinical data with a theoretical base.

Finally, Bowlby sees the reaction of the child as the abnormal rupture of an instinctual bond to the mother rather than a result of internalized aggression. Klaus and Kennell (1976) describe a similar "critical period" for emotional attachment in postpartum mothers and fathers. These authors believe that it is necessary for parents to have contact with their infant shortly after delivery for optimal development later. They postulate the formation of an innate bond during this period between parent and child which will continue for years. Klaus and Kennell support these speculations with animal research that demonstrates the ill effects of separating parents from neonates. The mother appears to lose interest in the infant and cannot give appropriate care if she is not present during this critical time.

In summary, depressive behavior has been observed in infants who are separated from their mothers. After a period of angry protest, these infants show unhappiness, withdrawal, and apathy. The question of whether this behavior is truly an example of depression, mourning, or a reaction to deprivation will be taken up in chapter 8.

Depression During Early Childhood

As a rule, children between the toddler years and the Oedipal phase appear to be remarkably free of depressive symptoms. In going over all the records of the outpatient department of the Children's Psychiatric Hospital at the University of Michigan Medical Center for a five-year period, Poznanski and Zrull (1970) found only one child under five years of age who could be considered as showing depressive symptoms. (Even with this child, the authors felt more confident in their diagnosis after a twoyear follow-up. This child exhibited a failure to thrive, quiet withdrawal, a fear of abandonment, and according to her mother, who rejected her, would show no affection toward anyone.)

Poznanski and Zrull comment on the gap in depressive symptoms between infancy and middle childhood, but conclude that they cannot account for it. They suggest that further study of the development of the preschooler's affects and drives is needed. On the other hand, the paucity of clinical reports of depression in this age group suggest to Poznanski and Zrull the question of whether it is possible for true affective disorders of clinical significance to occur in preschoolers or whether the manifestation of affective symptoms must await further maturation.

One possible explanation, which has been advanced by Anthony (1975) for the paucity of reports on childhood depression in general, is the young child's inability to verbalize how he feels. Depression must be inferred from the motor behavior of the young child and from his facial expressions, which is a difficult task. The motoric hyperactivity and general exuberance of the young child make him a poor candidate for a diagnosis of depression. Actually, as will be discussed later, the child's lack of verbal ability may lead to an overdiagnosis of depression since the examiner may tend to credit the child or infant with adult emotions and a more complex psychological make-up than is justified.

Mahler has closely observed children at this stage of development as part of her investigation of the separation-individuation process and has commented on the development of basic moods (1966) as well as on their behavioral manifestations. Mahler has not observed actual depressive symptoms in the early childhood stage, but she has noted behaviors that seem to indicate a predisposition to depression in later life. These predisposed children display excessive "separation and grief reactions marked by temper tantrums, continual attempts to woo or coerce the mother, and then giving up in despair for a while when unable to prevent separation" (1966, p. 163). Other evidence of this primary negative affective responsiveness consists of acts of impotent surrender and resignation, as well as discontentment and anger following a period of grief or sadness. In all cases Mahler found an increased clinging to the mother despite the lack of a truly satisfying relationship with her.

Mahler notes the volatility and transient nature of such moods, adding that such behaviors usually are seen only in context of the relationship with the mother and are absent when the child is alone or with others. She explains the presence of such activity by stressing the young child's disappointment in the mother and, secondarily, in the self. This disappointment prevents the full-length duration of the child's belief in the omnipotence of the mother which he requires for the development of his own sense of worth. The child shows a depletion of "confident expectation" from important others and suffers a subsequent diminution of self-esteem, which reduces the ability to neutralize aggression that later will account for the depressive symptoms. At this stage of development, however, depressive syndromes are not commonly seen, although (as will be discussed further in chapter 8) the groundwork for a predisposition to depression may be forming beneath the toddler's apparently exuberant and confident exterior.

Depression in Middle and Late Childhood

In recent years a number of articles have appeared describing depressive episodes, which phenomenologically resemble the adult syndromes, as occurring in older children (Poznanski and Zrull, 1970; Cytryn and McKnew, 1972; Weinberg et al., 1973; McConville et al., 1973). In the past such children were reported occasionally (Bierman et al., 1961) but they were considered to be clinical oddities or misdiagnosed. However, these reports did present fairly large series of children with apparently depressive symptoms, although the stringency of criteria for diagnosis varied from researcher to researcher. Another difficulty in assessing the true incidence of depression, even in older children, has been the proposing of "depressive equivalents" to exemplify the clinical expression of depression in childhood (Sperling, 1959; Toolan, 1962). The line of thinking that children express depression by certain ageappropriate equivalents has led to a plethora of clinical manifestations being diagnosed as forms of childhood affective disorders.

The terms "masked depression" or "depressive equivalents" appear to be somewhat confusing or inaccurate, since they have led to all sorts of symptoms being considered as evidence of depression. What may occur in some children is a depressed mood which is not sustained because the child cannot tolerate prolonged feelings of sadness or anguish. Some children lack the ability to bear depression and rapidly shift their attention to more pleasant thoughts or activities. There is still a sufficient fluidity between fantasy and reality so that harsh truths are avoided and general behavior is still directed by immediate pleasure, so that cognitive elements that produce depressive feelings are warded off and avoided. Therefore, some children are very capable of defending against depression by a variety of behaviors; however, their behaviors are not the equivalent of depression, nor are they evidence of a masked depression. Rather, their behaviors are adaptive attempts to deal with a situation which appears to the examiner as capable of evoking depression in an adult. If the child is forced to face his situation in a realistic manner, sadness may then be elicited. However, left to his own devices, a child may skillfully deny the realization of a depressing life situation, sometimes utilizing defenses against such a painful confrontation.

Hypomanic behaviors, hyperactivity, delinquency, and somatic complaints have been cited as defensive operations. Toolan (1962) further notes that male children or adolescents may feel ashamed of showing sadness or depression and cover these affects with forced joviality. Similarly, some cultural mores may sanction aggressive outbursts and ridicule a show of despair so that the former type of behavior is selected by the child.

This disparity in diagnostic criteria has led to highly variable reports of the incidence of depression in childhood. Annell (1971) compared the frequency with which different investigators made a diagnosis of depression and found that it ranged from 1.8 percent to 25 percent for all children seen. She correctly concluded that the main explanation for this marked variance was that different workers meant different things by depression. In spite of this confusion about the incidence of depression in middle childhood, an attempt will be made here to list some of the symptoms stressed by clinicians.

Weinberg et al. (1973) used a ten-symptom list to diagnose depression in their sample of children. In order to be so classified, a child had to show both a dysphoric mood and selfdepreciatory ideation, and at least two of the following eight symptoms: 1. aggressive behavior, 2. sleep disturbance, 3. a change in school performance, 4. diminished socialization, 5. change in attitude toward school, 6. somatic complaints, 7. loss of usual energy, and 8. unusual changes in appetite or weight.

Weinberg reported that forty-five of

seventy-two patients (aged six years, six months to twelve years, eight months) attending an educational guidance clinic met these criteria. His findings suggest a surprisingly high incidence of depression, although it may be that Weinberg selected an atypical group of children. He and his co-authors in fact mention that in half

of the children "depression" was considered secondary to learning or behavior problems, and perhaps was not a primary disorder.

In contrast, Poznanski and Zrull (1970) found only 14 depressed children of 1,788 children seen in their University of Michigan Medical Center study. These authors found the most frequent symptom to be a negative selfimage. Related symptoms were a fear of failure, the anticipation of unfair treatment, and feelings of inadequacy. A number of these children described themselves as bad. Overt signs were frequent crying and withdrawal. Sleep disturbances were less common than in nondepressed children. Aggressive behavior was evident in twelve of the fourteen depressed children, which led the authors to question the importance of inhibited, self-directed aggression as a significant psychodynamic of depression.

In an important theoretical paper, Sandler and Joffe (1965) also listed depressive symptoms they found in children undergoing psychiatric treatment: (1) The child appeared sad, unhappy, or depressed. (2) There was predominant withdrawal or lack of interest. (3) The child was discontented, with little capacity for pleasure. (4) The child communicated a sense of being unloved or rejected and turned away from disappointing others. (5) The child was not prepared to accept comfort. (6) There was a general tendency toward "oral passivity." (7) Insomnia or other sleep disturbance was noted. (8) Autoerotic or other repetitive activities were described. (9) It was difficult for the therapist to continue contact with the child. These authors were quick to point out that the children did not show these symptoms continuously and often the depressive aspect of their personalities formed part of another pathological syndrome. Other authors have not made these qualifying remarks. This difference in appreciation of the transient nature of symptoms may account for the great disparity in the reported incidence of depression in children. It is a rare child who is sad all the time and whose mood is not altered by novel situations. At the same time, almost all children show a temporary "depressed" mood in reaction to some external disappointments. Therefore, the diagnosis that is given depends on when the child is seen, whether the child is seen more than once, and whether the criteria for diagnosis require a sporadic or constant dysphoric mood.

In summarizing of the depressive symptoms of older children, the presence of a sad mood has been reported as well as a sense of withdrawal, disappointment, lack of relatedness, and overt aggression. Certain features of adult depression, however, usually are absent. There is no dread of the future, and no somatic symptoms such as psychomotor retardation or anorexia. The disorder also does not appear to be selfperpetuating or resistant to environmental variations. Children respond quickly to external changes and do not appear to sustain a prolonged sense of despair independently of life circumstances. Even among children at different stages of development, one would expect variation in the form of symptomatology which would be reflective of increasing cognitive growth.

McConville and his co-workers (1973) have noticed developmental variation in the type of depressive symptoms expressed by children of different ages. Their patient sample consisted of seventy-five children who were admitted to an inpatient psychiatric unit over a three-year period. Three types of depressive syndromes were observed. The "affectual" type was seen in children six to eight years of age and it primarily consisted of behavioral manifestations of sadness and helplessness. The "negative selfesteem" type consisted of verbalized feelings of worthlessness, of being unloved, and of being used by other people, and it was most commonly seen in the eight- to ten-year-old group. Finally a rare third type was called the "guilt" type because its prominent symptom was the child's conviction that he was wicked and should be dead or killed. This type was observed in the tento thirteen-year-old group. This study is significant; it demonstrates how even in middle to late childhood the normal developmental process can influence the expression of symptoms. The youngest children had difficulty verbalizing their feelings and their depression seemed to take the form of an overall sadness. The eight- to ten-year-olds could put their feelings into words and were able to identify states of self, but they did not as yet have a sense of inner evil. They continued to gauge their feelings as a response to others. Only as the children approached adolescence was there an internalization of some of the cognitive conditions for depression, the feeling of guilt and wickedness which justified the dysphoric state and perpetuated it despite environmental changes.

Illustrative Case History Of Depression In An Older Child

The example of the following child clinically illustrates severe depression in late childhood. Jimmy, an eleven-year-old boy, was seen after he wrote a series of pathetic, demanding notes to his parents. The notes were all repetitions of the same theme: that he was worthless and a failure and undeserving of their love, yet greatly needing their love. He had also asked his mother if it was a sin to commit suicide. The family history was remarkable in that the father had suffered from chronic depression since adolescence. He was a strict Catholic who constantly read inspirational books in search of a meaning in life. At home he was frequently unavailable, although he managed to put up a "good front" at his job. The father's side of the family had a high incidence of severe mental illness.

When seen for an evaluation, Jimmy was quiet and noncommunicative. He looked sad and was able to verbalize that he did not like himself. He stated that God had let him down and he was letting God down. When he was able to elaborate on this statement, he explained that he felt he had been born a poor athlete and a poor student, but he had not done his part by trying hard enough to overcome his innate deficiencies. He was totally convinced of his basic worthlessness, and furthermore he detested his weakness in not being able to overcome his alleged liabilities. Further contact revealed that because of his poor coordination, Jimmy was tormented by his peers and his brothers. He could find no area in his life in which he felt adequate or even safe. As a result of the excessively religious atmosphere at home, he believed that much of his misery was his own doing and he was a sinful creature because he gave in to feelings of failure. He also had been taught covertly to keep his feelings to himself and to be steadfast in the face of adversity. Actually, he felt like a little boy who wanted to be nurtured by his parents but he could not allow himself to express these longings openly. He felt overwhelmed by feelings of shame and inadequacy, but could not confide in anyone. He finally managed to allow these feelings to be partially communicated in his notes to his parents, although after writing them he refused to talk about their content with his mother or his father. Little Jimmy found himself in a desperate situation; he perceived himself as failing in what he believed his parents expected, but he could not bring himself to discuss his sense of frustration because of prior training. Similarly, he could not confess his terror of bullying peers. Instead he concluded that he was inferior. The more he suffered from his frustrations, the more he wanted nurturance at home, and the more he felt ashamed of his self-perceived infantile needs. He was a failure to himself, to his parents, and ultimately to God. He gradually began avoiding peers and stayed close to home. He lost interest in school and tried not to go by feigning illness. He withdrew, while being careful to look sad at dinner or when his family was present. Finally, he fortunately evoked a sympathetic response in his parents by his notes which initiated treatment and eventual recovery.

Attempts at Classification of Childhood Depression

Despite the theoretical debate over the possibility of true depression before adolescence, a few papers have appeared which take the occurrence of childhood depression as a clinical fact and attempt to classify these dysphoric states on such empirical grounds as response to treatment, the presence of precipitating events, or associated psychopathology.

Eva Frommer (1968) maintains that depression is quite common in childhood, accounting for 20 percent of all childhood psychopathology. She describes three major subgroups and one small additional grouping which may be a juvenile form of manicdepressive disorder. The first group is designated "enuretic depressive" because of the high incidence of bladder or bowel incontinence. In addition, these children exhibited learning disabilities and social withdrawal. Complaints of depression were present in only 19 percent of this group. Frommer states that treatment is prolonged and difficult, requiring more than antidepressant medication or group therapy. Removal from the home environment is sometimes indicated.

There is some question as to whether this group of children can actually be classified as depressed. They appear to be unfortunate and unhappy children who because of a combination of factors are neurologically immature and have learning disabilities and incontinence. Such children often get into chronic power struggles with their parents which increase their frustrations, but they do not appear depressed; rather, they are perpetually angry and resort to passive-aggressive retaliation against authority figures. They lack the negative self-image, the feeling of helplessness, and the blaming of self which appears necessary for the diagnosis of depression. Such children have been described adequately in the literature on enuresis, encopresis, or learning disabilities without reference to affective disorders.

Frommer's second major group is "uncomplicated depression." It is the largest group in her sample, and the children in it manifested irritability, weakness, and tendencies to recurrent explosions of temper. Half showed some sort of sleep disturbance and roughly onethird complained of feeling depressed. There was a lack of anxiety or decreased confidence. This group does appear to describe truly depressed children. After treatment there was significant academic improvement and others noted a change in the children's demeanor.

The third group was termed "phobic depressive" because of a high incidence of anxiety and a lack of confidence. Over two-thirds of these children exhibited abdominal pain or other somatic symptoms in order to stay home from school. Girls outnumbered boys by two to one in this group. Although Frommer calls such children depressed, they seem to fit the classic pattern of "school phobia." Gittleman Klein has recently studied a large group of such children and concludes that they are impaired by an abnormal persistence of separation anxiety so that they must stay near the mother figure. If they are allowed to remain with the mother, they are happy and relaxed. If they are forcibly separated, they exhibit panic and somatic symptoms. In neither situation are they depressed.

The last group described by Frommer are children with transient outbursts of temper alternating with periods of quiet reasonableness. She speculates rather cautiously that this group may be showing early symptoms of manic and depressive mood swings.

Frommer's work suffers from a lack of psychodynamic investigation as well as from her omission of the age ranges or developmental levels of her patients. However, the greatest drawback of her study is her overinclusion of nondepressed children in the depressive categories. Clinical depression entails more than situational unhappiness brought about by family conflicts, learning disabilities, or separation from parents.

A more profound and usable classification of depression in childhood has been presented by Cytryn and McKnew (1972). These authors differentiate between a depressive affectual response and a depressive illness, in which the depression is of long duration and the sad affect is associated with disturbance of vegetative functions or impairment of scholastic or social adjustment. In more severe cases, the child's thinking is said to be affected by feelings of despair, hopelessness, general retardation, and suicidal ideation. Having established these clear criteria of depressive illness, Cytryn and McKnew delineated three types of depressive disorders in children who ranged from six to twelve years of age.

The first type was classified as "masked depressive reaction" and was characterized by hyperactivity, aggressive behavior, psychosomatic illness, or delinquency. These children also exhibited periods of overt depression as well as depressive trends on psychological testing. The families of these children were chronically disorganized but showed no history of depression. If I understand the authors' concept of masked depression correctly, it is different from so-called depressive "equivalents." Cytryn and McKnew do not speculate that nondepressed behavior such as delinquency is a childhood expression of depression; rather, this behavior is seen as a defense against feeling depressed. Occasionally the defense breaks down and the underlying depression becomes manifest.

The second type was called "acute depressive reaction" and it resulted from a clearly identifiable environmental cause, usually invoking the loss of the attention of a loved one. These children exhibited clear symptoms of depression for a short period of time and then recovered quickly. There was usually a history of good premorbid adjustment and their families demonstrated considerable strength and cohesion as well as an absence of depression. It might be difficult to separate such children from those exhibiting a grief or mourning reaction. It is speculated that the child's defenses are momentarily shaken but that reconstitution usually follows unless there are persistent environmental traumas.

Finally, they described a more severe "chronic depressive reaction" in which there was no history of a precipitating event. These children did not reconstitute rapidly and showed evidence of long-standing depression. There was a history of repeated separation from loved ones and deprivation beginning early in life. All of these children had at least one parent who suffered from recurrent depression.

This last group supports the findings of Poznanski and Zrull (1970) that the depression of the children they studied was not reactive to an immediate trauma, but part of an ongoing life process. They also found a high incidence of parental depression, frequent harsh treatment of the child, and overt parental rejection. It would appear that Poznanski and Zrull are describing the "chronic" type of child in Cytryn and McKnew's classification. The former authors may have set more stringent criteria for the diagnosis of depression and excluded those children classified as having "masked" or "acute" depression by Cytryn and McKnew. The possible merit of this more narrow definition of depression is that it allows for a study of the natural history of the disorder by excluding children whose depressive symptoms may be part of a transient grief reaction, or submerged beneath delinquent activity or other defenses. For example, in an important follow-up study Poznanski, Krahenbuhl, and Zrull (1976) found that half of their original sample (now in adolescence) was still depressed. An additional finding was that the childhood aggression had diminished and pathological dependency, common in adult depression, was more prominent. Among the patients who were still depressed, the pattern of parental rejection and deprivation had continued. It can be hypothesized that in these cases, the causes of depression became internalized and adequate coping mechanisms were prevented from crystallizing. On the other hand, it may equally be speculated that the "masked" type of depression described by Cytryn and McKnew would eventually follow a delinquent career and the "acute" type would not show pathology in adolescence.

Perhaps a follow-up study by these authors will clarify these questions as well as justify labeling children as depressed who are able to defend against depression or exhibit a transient state of grief over an environmental trauma. The theoretical problem (to be considered in chapter 8) is whether children who do not exhibit prolonged depression can be truly classified as suffering from a depressive illness. Children who exhibit equivalent or masked depressions may not be actually depressed. Rather, the examiner may infer that they should be depressed because of their difficult life circumstances. If these children can muster defenses against adverse environmental situations, then there may be a question as to whether they should be considered to be suffering from depression.

Taking these problems into consideration, Malmquist (1971) has attempted an allencompassing diagnostic classification based simply on the predominance of depressive affect. He includes criteria of different conceptual levels, such as descriptive clinical features, age, and etiology. His classification is presented in Table 4-1.

Malmquist arrived at this classification by an exhaustive review of the literature. His system is extremely valuable in briefly presenting all of the possible states that have been called depression in children. His classification, reproduced here as Table 4-1, can be taken as a summary of current knowledge of the symptomatic picture of childhood and adolescent depression. The reader is free to agree or disagree with the inclusion of certain subgroups, but all are essentially reported by Malmquist. The common thread of depressive affect[8] as the sole criterion for diagnosing depression cuts across theoretical differences but may ultimately be misleading since, as mentioned, a sad affect can be seen in numerous non-depressive conditions.

Table 4-1

Classification of Childhood Depressions

I. Associated with Organic Diseases

A. Part of Pathologic Process

1. Leukemia

2. Degenerative Diseases 3.

Infectious Diseases
4. Metabolic Diseases—Pituitary Disease, Juvenile Diabetes, Thyroid Disease, etc.

5. Nutritional or Vitamin Deficiency States

B. Secondary (Reactive) to a Physical Process

II. Deprivation syndromes: Reality-Based Reactions to Impoverished or Nonrewarding Environment

A. Anaclitic Depressions

B. "Affectionless" Character Types

III. Syndromes Associated with Difficulties in Individuation

A. Problems of Separation-Individuation

B. School Phobias with Depressive Components

C. Developmental Precursors of "Moral Masochism"

IV. Latency Types

A. Associated with Object Loss
B. Failure to Meet Unattainable Ideals
C. "Depressive Equivalents" (Depression without Depressive Affect)

   1. Somatization (Hypochondriacal Patterns)

   2. Hyperkinesis
   3. Acting Out

   4. Delayed Depressive Reactions

      a. Mourning at Distance
      b. Overidealization Processes Postponing Reaction
      c. Denial Patterns

   5. Eating Disturbances (Obesity Syndromes)

D. Manic-Depressive States

E. "Affectless" Character Types (Generalized Anhedonia)

F. Obsessional Character (Compensated Depressive)

V. Adolescent Types

    A. Mood Lability as Developmental Process

    B. Reactive to Current Loss

    C. Unresolved Mourning from Current Losses

    D. Earlier Losses ("Trauma") Now Dealt with by Ego

    E. Acting-Out Depressions

    F. Schizophrenias with Prominent Affective Components

    G. Continuation of Earlier Types (I, IV)

Source: From "Depression in Childhood and Adolescence" by C. Malmquist, *New England Journal of Medicine* 284 (1971). Reprinted by permission.

This section must end on a note of frustration and an admission of incompleteness. As yet there is no adequate classification of depression in childhood, nor are there any agreed criteria for the diagnosis of depression before adolescence. It seems almost plausible to base a classification on the developmental process as McConville (1973) tentatively attempted. Children are limited by their cognitive and affective capacities in their ability to experience and express feelings of depression. What elicits depression also obviously changes as the child matures. Young infants do not have problems of self-esteem, just as preschoolers cannot be said to be haunted by a fear of a deprived future. Ultimately the question of childhood depression may be solved as our knowledge of normal development increases.

Depression in Adolescence

In contrast to the questionable existence of depression in childhood, there is little doubt that depression definitely is experienced by adolescents. The difficulty with this stage of development is that depression may be too ubiquitous. The normal mood swings of the adolescent may give the impression of an epidemic of depressive disorders occurring after puberty. The problem is in differentiating the truly depressed youngster from the normally moody adolescent who is showing transient episodes of dysphoric affect as an overreaction to relatively trivial disappointments. Jacobson (1961) has investigated the causes for the adolescent's moodiness and she believes that emotional lability is a manifestation of a remodeling of the individual's psychic structure secondary to massive biological, social, and psychological changes. Jacobson views adolescence as a time when the individual must break with ties from the past (including old identifications with adult figures) to forge a new image of the self. The individual is pressured by both the id and the superego in the formation of a new identity, leading to alternating periods of sexual and aggressive acting out; repentant, moralistic behavior; as well as feelings of guilt, shame, and inferiority. According to Jacobson the ego does not gain sufficient stability until late adolescence so that, in the first few years following puberty, there are bound to be mood swings reflecting the dominance of id or superego forces over a relatively weak ego. Depression may be experienced as part of adolescent development for additional reasons: the relinquishing of childhood ties and pursuits, the failure to live up to unrealistic ideals, and as the result of guilt conflicts. Jacobson views adolescence as a turbulent time, with extensive psychic alterations, mood swings, and transient depression to be expected.

Other authors (Weiner, 1970) have disagreed with the view that adolescence must be a stage of turmoil and emotional lability. Disturbed adolescence is not the rule, but is the result of a disturbed childhood and the forerunner of disturbed maturity. This debate goes beyond the scope of this work but in my opinion the truth is somewhere between these two positions. The clinical literature based on severely disturbed adolescents probably has been too generously applied to all adolescents. Also, the cultural milieu may greatly affect the turbulence of adolescence. Certainly not all adolescents go through the painful traumas described by some authors. For some individuals this is not only a peaceful but a very satisfying time of life. Nevertheless, our own culture places the adolescent under a great deal of stress in terms of sexual inhibition, limitations of freedom, pressure for social and academic success, and a lack of a definable cultural role, so that disturbed behavior is not surprising.

There is also a lack of maturity of judgment that affects the adolescent, regardless of cultural milieu that may predispose him to impulsive acts and inappropriately extreme reactions. As pertaining to depression, some adolescents present such an air of urgency and total despair, as well as an alarming tendency toward self destructive acts, that a more malignant schizophrenic process is suspected. Some adolescents become extremely agitated and others withdraw from all contact with peers. One youngster, for example, spent days alone in his room with blankets over his face while listening to records, and he refused to take meals or talk with his family. There is also an unrealistic sense of finality in the thinking of some adolescents; failure to make the school honor role means that one will be marked for life as a failure, or rejection by a peer means that one will never be acceptable to others. This lack of perspective makes the symptoms more severe and more dangerous. A related quality of cognition in some adolescents is a lack of moderation. People, society, or they themselves are all good or all bad, depending on most recent experience. One very bright fourteen-year-old boy who had been disappointed by the treatment others accorded him in his first few days of high school spent his first session on a long tirade about the innate evil of mankind and the dehumanizing effects of a materialistic society. His erudite argument was motivated by his not being given the deference he thought he deserved. Within a few weeks, after he had adjusted to his new surroundings, the world became benevolent and capitalism was now a viable system of economics. Fortunately many of these adolescent depressions are characterized by their brevity as much as by their intensity.

Other depressions, however, become chronic and no longer respond to an amelioration of external circumstances. These youngsters present depressive symptoms similar to those found in adult patients, or they may present age-specific defenses against depression. Among these defenses are restlessness, drug use, group affiliation, delinquency, or sexual promiscuity. Easson (1977) has reviewed the myriad defenses against depression in adolescence and related each to the underlying causes of a painful affect. Self-contempt may result in rebelliousness, drug use, or aggressive acts. Depression resulting from frustration of dependency needs may produce agitation, anxiety, and a desperate need to substitute new gratifying figures for the lost parents, leading to joining a gang or indiscriminate sexual unions.

Illustrative Case History Of Depression In A Young Adolescent

The following clinical vignette is

representative of a fairly severe depressive illness in a young teenager. Betty, a fifteen-yearold girl, came for treatment after suddenly experiencing a crying spell in school. Following this outburst she refused to return to school, where she was an honor student. When seen for an evaluation Betty looked sad and lifeless with occasional tears in her eyes. She also complained of nausea and a choking sensation. She felt that she wanted to hurt herself because she was a failure, she was ugly, and she had humiliated herself in front of her schoolmates by weeping. She believed she could never become a model as she had desired to be, because she was not sufficiently pretty or poised. In actuality she was a very attractive young girl. She exuded a sense of quiet panic over being unable to control her painful feelings. There was no sleep disturbance but Betty was plagued by dreams in which she felt lost and alone or in which strange people were chasing her.

Further history revealed that Betty had not let herself enjoy anything for the past year. The reasons for her enforced anhedonia were that she felt unworthy because she sensed herself to be a disappointment to her mother as well as to herself. She began experiencing feelings of depression after she met a boy at a summer resort. She wanted the boy to pursue her but she also felt guilty about her romantic desires. The boy did not follow through and this convinced her that she was ugly and undesirable. She also hinted that this "rejection" was well deserved because she should have devoted herself only to her studies and her family. Since this episode she constantly began to evaluate both herself and the way others treated her. Mild snubs were magnified and remembered until she felt uniformly disliked. She started hating to go to school which had become a source of alleged belittling.

Betty's mother was a very disturbed woman who resented her familial role. She had pushed Betty into nursery school despite protests and later forced her to go to sleep-away camp. She was constantly critical of everyone and pictured herself as a martyr to her family. The father withdrew into his business and seemed to avoid coming home. The only praise Betty ever received was for her academic success, but even this pleasure was destroyed by the mother's use of her daughter's grades to degrade her other children.

Betty had never truly developed a sure sense of her own worth but relied excessively on her mother's opinions. She cherished normal adolescent romantic notions which she kept secret. When these dreams were dashed by her supposed "rejection," she erroneously believed that her secret desires would never be fulfilled, and she would always be unworthy and unlovable, just as her mother had covertly predicted. Only one experience appeared sufficient to convince her of the inevitability of a terrible fate. From that point on she unconsciously distorted the reactions of others to reaffirm her unworthiness and she selected only those responses that confirmed her low opinion of herself. Gradually her affective state deteriorated in step with her unconscious cognitive beliefs and culminated in a severe depression.

Juvenile Manic-Depressive Disorders

If the clinical status of depression in childhood is problematic, the occurrence of manic-depressive disorders before puberty is even more questionable. Kraepelin (1921) noted that a few of his adult manic-depressive patients reported experiencing their first episode before age ten, one patient as early as age five. Other investigators also have described adult patients who traced their illness back to early childhood; however, actual observed case reports of manicdepressive disorder before puberty are rare.

In the late nineteenth century and in the early part of this century, alleged cases of childhood mania were reported (see Anthony and Scott, 1960, for a detailed review) but it remains doubtful that these children were truly manic. Any cyclical behavior or period of excitement seems to have been diagnosed as mania. A close reading of these early reports is needed, since the present-day syndrome of minimal brain dysfunction—which predominantly consists of hyperactivity, distractibility, and emotional lability—could have been confused with manic behavior. Since these symptoms depend on the amount of external stimulation, the condition could have appeared to be episodic or cyclical. Therefore it is debatable whether these early reports were actually describing hyperactive rather than manic children. When Anthony and Scott reviewed twenty-eight such case reports, applying fairly rigorous criteria for the diagnosis of manic-depressive illness, they found only three reported children who met over five of their ten criteria, and none scored over seven. All three children were eleven years old and showed alternation of depression and mania. Anthony and Scott believe that "all the other cases were open to the charge of misdiagnosis" (1960, p. 58). This conclusion fits the earlier findings of Kasanin and Kaufman (1929) that affective psychoses do not occur in early childhood. These authors reviewed 6,000 patients and found that in only four cases an affective psychosis began before age sixteen and never before age fourteen.

Despite this somewhat uncertain position on the possibility of manic-depressive illness in childhood, some cases have been reported, especially since the discovery of the effectiveness of lithium for treating this disorder. Anthony and Scott (1960) reported the case of a twelve-yearold boy who was seen with symptoms of acute mania which subsided and then returned. This boy's history was recorded up to the time he was twenty-two years old. By then he had been hospitalized four times with a clear-cut manicdepressive disorder. The authors emphasized that the illness began before puberty. They concluded that although manic-depressive disorders are clinically rare in childhood, they are psychodynamically possible because children may utilize grandiose fantasies as a defense against feelings of sadness or disappointment.

Since the appearance of this paper, other authors have presented single case histories of manic attacks in young adolescents (Warneke, 1975; Berg, Hullin, and Allsopp, 1974). Although it is of clinical interest as well as therapeutic importance that lithium was successfully used in these cases, the articles merely call attention to a few rare cases of manic-depressive illness which began in adolescence. However, two articles have reported manic episodes in very young children, therefore tending to justify this disorder as a bona fide pediatric illness. The first article by Feinstein and Wolpert (1973) speculates that certain children may show precursors of later manic-depressive behavior. They report the case of a three-and-one-halfyear-old girl with a strong family history of this disorder who began to show rapid mood alterations from the age of two. She eventually was seen because of hyperactivity and distractibility. Later she is described as reacting to an alleged disappointment with prolonged agitation and destructive behavior. (Her sister had accompanied her to the psychiatric appointment, although simply to see another psychiatrist who shared the same waiting room.) Due to the child's extreme aggressive behavior, she was tried on lithium at age five and one-half, with good effect. There was no recurrence of her agitation or destructiveness. On the basis of her family history, the episodes of hyperactivity, and her response to lithium, the authors conclude that their patient is an example of juvenile manic-depressive illness. They doubt that the hyperactivity was the consequence of minimal brain dysfunction since this form of hyperactivity is unresponsive to lithium.

Thompson and Schindler (1976) describe a five-year-old boy who was seen because of a short attention span, wandering thoughts, and disruptive classroom behavior. Past history was significant in that the child had been abandoned by his parents and spent a deprived infancy, possibly with nutritional deficiency, in an orphanage. At age three he was adopted by loving parents who showered the boy with care and attention. On evaluation there were no neurological findings, despite his distractibility. He was jovial and showed a constantly elevated mood. The authors speculate that the boy's exuberant behavior may have resulted from his sudden favorable circumstances—being placed in a loving and giving environment after having been raised in the deprivation of a poorly run orphanage. His separation from this allrewarding environment when he started school may have set off fears of loss and a return to deprivation which, according to the authors, led to his increasing manic behavior.

These two reports are certainly provocative but they leave crucial questions unanswered. There was no alternation of so-called manic behavior with states of depression, which would have truly confirmed the diagnosis. Furthermore, the manic behavior itself consisted of hyperactivity, distractibility, grandiose fantasies, and in one case aggressive behavior. A difficulty not mentioned is that such behavior is common in many children who have variations of minimal brain dysfunction. Grandiose fantasies also are a fairly normal method of defense in all young children who confuse fantasy and reality in their attempts to compensate for being small and socially powerless. The same argument can be leveled at Anthony and Scott's claim that the psychodynamics of manic depression may be found in children. This is certainly true, for children are realistically dependent on others, have difficulty resolving ambivalence, and are prone to an omnipotent denial of reality. These psychodynamic characteristics are found in normal children who do not show features of affective disorders. Therefore the presence of such psychodynamics may be a necessary but not sufficient cause for the expression of manicdepressive behavior. The point is that these authors do not demonstrate, either on a clinical or psychodynamic basis, the specificity needed to make this diagnosis. The child who improved on lithium may be cited as showing some form of specificity in terms of drug response. However, lithium has been tried in a variety of childhood disorders, especially aggressive behavior, with reportedly good effects (Annell, 1969) so that its effects may not be that specific for manicdepressive disorders. The speculation that a childhood predisposition to manic-depressive disorders does exist nevertheless is an extremely intriguing proposition. This predisposition may take the form of excessive affective lability or impulsivity which, given a sufficiently pathological home environment and a precipitating trauma, may ultimately result in a cyclical illness. Proving the existence of such susceptibility, however, must await comparison studies of children from highly affected families, who are either raised with their natural parents or have been adopted in early infancy by normal parents so that they do not grow up subjected to their parents' cyclical moods.

Conclusion

This chapter has reviewed the clinical syndromes that have been called depression in children. There is still much controversy whether true depression can exist prior to late childhood. The reaction of infants to separation may be better conceived of as a grief reaction, and the transient unhappy moods of the young child may be considered a direct, behavioral reaction to momentary disappointments. Even when states similar to adult depression are manifested in later childhood, the symptoms are influenced by the appropriate cognitive and affective developmental level. The pendulum of psychiatric opinion has swung back and forth as to whether depression in childhood exists, but this continuing argument may ultimately center on a semantic difference: the question is not whether depression exists in childhood, but rather how the developmental process allows or limits the experience or expression of varying pathological moods and affects.

Notes

[8] Malmquist also includes "depressive equivalents."

PART TWO

Psychodynamics

[5]

THE PSYCHOBIOLOGY OF

SADNESS

Silvano Arieti

Introductory Remarks

Many psychiatrists warn the therapist in training not to confuse sadness, or normal unhappiness, with depression. The warning is appropriate, but certainly the confusion would not arise if there were no similarities between these two human conditions. And even if the similarities were less important than the differences, they would deserve to be studied, unless proved coincidental or casual.

In many scientific fields progress is often made when two or more conditions or things which are apparently alike can be differentiated and eventually proved dissimilar in their basic structure. But progress on many occasions is made also in the opposite way, when similarities appearing in different conditions are recognized as not being casual, adventitious, or coincidental, but indications of relatedness between the nature of the phenomena involved. As a matter of fact, in some cases one of the two similar conditions is fundamentally only a quantitative transformation of the other. For instance, fever is different from normal body temperature, but it is nevertheless a body temperature raised by some special contingencies.

I believe that a close relation exists between sadness, a normal emotion, and depression, which is a psychiatric symptom or condition. Undoubtedly I am predisposed to think so by some personal bias, but I am aware of the opposite bias held by most authors who see a completely different nature in sadness and depression. These authors interpret depression only or almost exclusively as a chemical event occurring in the brain. I do not deny that a chemical event occurs in the brain when people experience depression. In fact, I believe that a chemical event occurs even when they experience sadness. But the chemical event is an effect, and to some extent the medium of the psychological event, with which I—as a psychiatrist, psychologist, or therapist—am mainly concerned. The psychological event may be caused by an external event or by a previous psychological event, or a combination of the two, and it has to be studied by me, a psychotherapist, as such. Naturally I do not disregard or consider useless the study of the neuronal and biochemical events which necessarily accompany the psychological event. If in the experience of these phenomena we recognize the primacy of the psychological event, I believe it then will be easier to recognize a relation between normal sadness and abnormal depression.

When a normal person is sad or unhappy as a result of some unpleasant events which have occurred in his life, at times he calls himself depressed and melancholy. Similarly we may call our most depressed psychiatric patients sad, melancholy, anguished, unhappy. This free interchange of adjectives is based on the fact that all of them imply a similar feeling of "unpleasure." Perhaps we could bypass the study of sadness and proceed directly to the study of the syndrome called depression if we knew all there is to know about sadness, but unfortunately this is far from being the case. In the indexes of many major books on depression, I found no entry for such items as sadness and unhappiness. Sadness and unhappiness also do not appear in the psychological dictionary by English and English (1958), the psychiatric dictionary by Hinsie and Campbell (1960), and the *Dictionary of Behavioral Science* by Wolman (1973).

Normal sadness is the emotional effect on a human being when he apprehends a situation that he would have preferred not to occur, and which he considers adverse to his well-being. This definition would not pass the test of a rigorous logician. It is to some extent circular, like all definitions that refer to the subjective life of the individual, and it shows once again our difficulty in overcoming the mind-body dichotomy. Nevertheless I think we can use it as a working definition.

First we must remember that sadness presupposes the capacity to experience other normal emotions and conditions, such as affection, closeness, love, self-respect, feelings of satisfaction. In fact, the lack or loss of these positive emotions makes us vulnerable to sadness.

Sadness has many characteristics similar to other feelings and emotions, as well as some special traits of its own. Before taking sadness as the object of our study, we will review some aspects of all feelings. This is an unusual procedure in psychiatric books; but feelings do pertain to all psychiatric conditions and in particular to affective disorders. Studying them, even as they occur in nonpathological conditions, seems to me an essential prerequisite not only for psychological but also for psychiatric studies.

Feelings And Experiences Of Inner Status[9]

In the English language the word feeling can refer to all subjective or private experiences from elementary sensations to complicated emotions.

Sensations, when they reach the level of perceptions, have two experiential aspects: they consist of a subjective apprehension of a physical state of the organism (for instance, a specific unpleasant feeling which we call pain), and they mirror an aspect of reality.

One aspect is sensory, or the transformation of a bodily change into an experience of an inner status, an experience that as a subjective event occurs within the organism. On the other side we have the function of mirroring reality, a function which generally expands into numerous ramifications that have to do with cognition.

If we examine sensory perceptions, we recognize that the importance of these two components varies tremendously. The experience of inner status is very important in the perception of pain, hunger, thirst, and temperature. It becomes less pronounced in other perceptions when the organism is of necessity in contact with some stimuli (tactile, gustatory, and, less obviously, olfactory) coming from the external world. In these perceptions the subjective alteration of the organism plays the predominant role, but the presence of the

external stimulus generally also is acknowledged.

In auditory and visual perceptions, the experience of a change of inner status plays a minimal role. What is most important is the awareness these perceptions give us of what happens in the external world; thus they enable the organism to deal more appropriately with the world. They are to a great extent the foundation of cognition, they develop connections with the symbolism of language, they are elaborated to the level of apperception, and they become increasingly removed from their sensorial origin. Their importance finally no longer lies in their sensorial nature but in their meaning.

Both kinds of experience are purposeful, but the experiences of inner status have an immediate survival value and are fundamentally not symbolic, and the experiences of mirroring of reality soon acquire a symbolic function and have less immediate survival value.

I must point out that I have oversimplified this complex matter for expository reasons. No experience, especially at a human level, is ever exclusively of one type or another, but only predominantly of one type. Although in this chapter we are particularly interested in the experiences of inner status, I shall make a few remarks about the general character of cognitive experiences in order to highlight their differences from the experiences of inner status.

Cognitive experiences become symbolic, that is, they acquire the property of making things stand for other things. For instance, sounds stand for words, things, and meanings.

Therefore this field of cognition becomes potentially endless. It is a constantly enlarging system which must be fully evaluated as a capacity of the individual, as a social and a historical phenomenon in the spatial dimension of the community, and in the temporal dimension of the history of man. Symbols are created continuously and they become more and more detached from their original perceptual foundation. What starts as a simple perception continues as a probe of wider and wider horizons. The finitude of man seems temporarily overcome by the use of the symbolic process.

In contrast to this unlimited scope, it at first seems that the experiences of inner status play only a secondary role, at least in the human organism. They cannot expand endlessly and they seem by necessity concerned with hereand-now reality, a reality restricted to the boundaries of the organism, but one which immediately can be divided into pleasant and unpleasant experiences.

Has the organism really relegated the experiences of inner status to a secondary role? Not at all, as will be apparent if in paradigmatic fashion we take into consideration one of these experiences: an unpleasant one, pain.

When some special nerve endings are stimulated, there is a flow of stimulation which eventually reaches the thalamus and the cerebral cortex, and pain is experienced. Pain is not just a sensation and a perception. It is a warning, a signal that a discontinuity or an adverse change has occurred in the body, which may persist and increase unless the organism removes the source of pain. Pain thus translates an abnormal state of the animal organism into a subjective experience. Lower species attempt to remove pain by motor withdrawal from its source. Higher species and especially human beings generally attempt to remove the source of pain by purposeful behavior so that the regenerative potential of the organism can permit healing. If we have a toothache, we rush to the dentist.

But long before we have the capacity to understand the meaning of a toothache and to seek the help of a dentist, we have the capacity to understand pain. The baby has such a capacity in his very first day of life. Pain for him is an immediate revelation antecedent to any learning. The subjective unpleasant experience is instantaneous. It operates prior to and much faster than any cognitive experience that derives from the elaboration of the second type of sensations—perceptions. The baby does not know how to talk but he is able to express his experience of pain by crying. The fact that he cries tells us that he is already capable of attributing a negative *value* to pain. The baby seems also to convey a message to the adult: "Remove my pain by feeding me, holding me, changing my clothes."

When the child gets older, he does not cry anymore but the motivation is the same: "Remove the source of pain." This removal is attempted with the help of others or by one's own efforts. Thus the value—in this case negative—which is immediately perceived even by the infant as inherent in a particular state of awareness, corresponds to an objective value for life in general and promotes a special type of motivated behavior. In other words, the feeling of pain becomes a motivational force, and the motivation is to eliminate the source of the pain, or at least to give a warning that a method should be found to eliminate the cause of that feeling.

Of course there is no perfect

correspondence between the intensity of the painful feeling, the warning implied, and the resulting behavior. A toothache can cause very distressing pain and a serious disease may produce only a dull pain. In some serious diseases the pain becomes noticeable or unbearable when the illness has reached an advanced degree which may be beyond remedy at the present stage of our therapeutic knowledge. Even if the system of feeling pain is not a precise signaling equipment or a sophisticated diagnostician, in its total effect it is of tremendous and indispensable value for the organism. It is logical to assume that pain was at first selected in evolution because the animal, unlike vegetable life, moves or changes positions and needs a sensation signal to avoid surrounding bodies having certain harmful characteristics (too hard, cutting edges, thorns, etc.). Pain is also an indicator, although an imperfect one, of certain internal harmful states and diseases of the organism. We can assume safely that pain perception has such a survival value that without it animal life would not be possible, except for the simplest species.

Elsewhere (Arieti, 1960, 1967) I have described how emotions share some of the properties of simple feelings, such as sensations and perceptions of inner status. Emotions too can be divided into those that are pleasant and unpleasant and therefore they become motivational forces: pleasant emotions motivate a behavior aimed at preserving the pleasure, and unpleasant emotions motivate a behavior aimed at ending the unpleasantness. What Freud called cathexis—that is, investment of energy or libido —is probably only the motivational value of felt experiences, as Freud himself thought before he wrote *The Ego and the Id.*

We must carefully take into consideration two important issues concerning emotions.

Many well-known psychologists (for instance, Woodworth, 1940; Munn, 1946) have considered emotions as a disorganization of the organism. It is to the merit of Leeper (1948) that he showed the fallacy of this position. I myself have independently pursued the line initiated by Leeper, and I have described the highly organized status of emotions and their motivations (Arieti, 1960, 1967). For instance, a state of tension is motivationally organized to induce a return to homeostasis and a state of satisfaction, fear warns us of a present danger and prepares us to cope with it, anxiety warns us against a future or indefinite danger, rage and anger put us in a position to fight an adverse force, and so on. The experience of emotion is indeed a change in the organism and thus may be a disturbance, but not a disorganization.

The second characteristic, which I described fully for the first time in *The Intrapsychic Self* (1967), consists of the fact that at a human level all emotions have a cognitive component, minimal in some emotions and preponderant in others.

Emotions can be divided into three orders or ranks (Arieti, 1967, 1970a, 1970b). The first rank includes the simplest emotions which I have called first-order or protoemotions. There are at least five types: (1) tension, a feeling of discomfort caused, for example, by excessive stimulation and hindered physiological or instinctual response; (2) appetite, a feeling of expectancy which accompanies a tendency to move toward, contact, grab, or incorporate an almost immediately attainable goal; (3) fear, an unpleasant subjective state which follows the perception of danger and elicits a readiness to flee; (4) rage, an emotion that follows the perception of a danger to be overcome by fighting; that is, by aggressive behavior rather than by flight; (5) satisfaction, an emotional state resulting from gratification of physical needs and relief from other emotions.

In a general sense we can say about protoemotions that: (1) They are experiences of inner status which cannot be sharply localized and which involve the whole or a large part of the organism. (2) They either include a set of bodily changes, mostly muscular and humoral, or retain some bodily characteristics. (3) They are elicited by the presence or absence of specific stimuli which are perceived by the organism to be related in a positive or negative way to its safety and comfort. (4) They become important motivational factors and to a large extent determine the type of external behavior of the subject. (5) They have an almost immediate effect; if they unchain a delayed reaction, the delay ranges from a fraction of a second to a few minutes. (6) In order to be experienced, they require a minimum of cognitive effort. For instance in fear or rage a stimulus must promptly be recognized as a sign of danger. The danger is present or imminent.

The fifth and sixth characteristics require further discussion. Protoemotions are not experienced instantaneously, like the simple sensations of pain and thirst. They require some cognitive work. However, this cognitive work is of very short duration and presymbolic, or in some cases symbolic to a rudimentary degree. Presymbolic cognition includes perception and simple learning. It also includes the sensorimotor intelligence described by Piaget in the first year and a half of life.

Protoemotions are extremely important for the survival of the species and also as motivational forces. They are important in both infrahumans and man. However, let us remember that the learning which is required at this level is very simple. It deals with messages immediately given with either direct stimuli or signals, but not with symbols. Signals or signs indicate things. Some of them may actually be parts of things. (The smell of a mouse is connected to or part of the mouse for the cat.) However, they are not necessarily so. Like the ringing of a bell for the conditioned dog, they indicate something which is forthcoming.

Organization at the protoemotional level is

very simple. It does not include what is most pertinent in the field of psychiatry. In fact, we must go to the second-order emotions to find such psychological experiences as anxiety, anger, wishing, security.

Second-order emotions are not elicited by a direct or impending attack or by a threatened immediate change in homeostasis of the organism, but by cognitive symbolic processes. The prerequisite learning deals not only with immediate stimuli or signals, but also with symbols; that is, with something which represents stimuli or stands for the direct sensedata.

These symbols may vary from very simple forms to the most complicated and abstract representations. The simplest symbol is the image, a psychological phenomenon which has been badly neglected in psychology and psychiatry. We know that an image is a memory trace which assumes the form of a representation. It is an internal quasireproduction of a perception that does not require the corresponding external stimulus in order to be evoked. Although we cannot deny that at least rudimentary images occur in subhuman animals, there seems to be no doubt that images are predominantly a human characteristic. The child closes his eyes and visualizes his mother. The mother may not be present, but her image is with the child and it stands for her. He may lie peacefully in bed and that image will be with him until he falls asleep. By the image representing her, the mother acquires a psychic reality which is not tied to her physical presence.

Image formation is actually the basis for all higher mental processes. It enables the human being not only to re-evoke what is not present, but to retain an affective disposition for the absent object. The image thus becomes a substitute for the external object. It is actually an inner object, although it is not well organized.

Now let us see how images may increase the emotional gamut. Anxiety is the emotional reaction to the expectation of danger. The danger is not immediate, nor is it always well defined. The expectation of danger is not the result of a simple perception or signal, as it is in the case of fear. Images enable the person to anticipate a future danger and its dreaded consequences, even though he does not expect it to materialize for some time. In its simplest form anxiety is fear mediated by images or imagined fear. However, often the danger is represented by sets of symbols which are more complicated than sequences of images.

Similar remarks could be made for the other second-order emotion, anger. In its simplest form anger is imagined rage; that is, a rage elicited by the images of the stimuli which generally elicit rage. Whereas rage usually leads to immediate motor discharge directed against the stimulus that elicits it, anger tends to last longer although it retains an impelling characteristic. The prolongation of anger is possible because it is mediated by symbolic forms, just as anxiety is. If rage was useful for survival in the jungle, anger was useful for the first human communities to maintain a hostiledefensive attitude toward the enemy, even when the latter was not present.

Wishing is an emotional state which has received little consideration in psychology except when it has been confused with appetite. Whereas appetite is a feeling accompanied by a preparation of the body for approach and incorporation, wishing means a pleasant attraction toward something or somebody, or toward doing something. Contrary to appetite, wishing is made possible by the evocation of the image or other symbols of an object whose presence is pleasant. The image of an earlier

pleasant experience—for instance, the satisfaction of a need—evokes an emotional disposition which motivates the individual to replace the image with the real object of satisfaction. A search for the real object thus is initiated or at least contemplated. This search may require detours, since a direct approach is often not possible.

Security is the last second-order emotion. It has played an important role in the theoretical framework of the psychiatrist Harry Stack Sullivan (1940, 1953). It is debatable whether such an emotion really exists; the term may indicate only the absence of unpleasant emotions or else be a purely hypothetical concept. We can visualize the simplest form of security as imagined satisfaction. That is, images permit the individual to visualize a state of satisfaction not only for today but also for tomorrow.

The brain, which uses images, can be compared to some extent to an analog computer.

With the advent of language, the nervous system in some aspects becomes like a digital computer; a system of arbitrary signs is now capable of eliciting the emotions that earlier could be engendered only by external stimuli or images. Until now emotions seem to be only experiences of inner states which are connected with the organism itself, its immediate surroundings, or its image of the immediate surroundings. Emotions, as experiences of inner states and with some exceptions to be discussed later, are not symbolic. They stand only for themselves and they do not extend beyond the boundaries of the organism. However, when they become connected with symbolism, they are capable of partaking of the infinity of the universe.

Second-order emotions can be elicited also by a preconceptual type of cognition; that is, by primitive forms of thinking included in what Freud called the primary process. The nonhuman animal is at a level where only first-order emotions are possible and so is very limited psychologically; it remains within the boundaries of a limited reality but is indeed a realist. It is capable only of a nonsymbolic type of learning. It interprets signs but not symbols in the light of past experience. When man uses symbols, especially preconceptual symbols, he opens his mind toward the infinity of the universe but also toward an infinity of errors and the realm of unreality. For instance, the experience of anxiety may be wasted because it is based not on a realistic appreciation of danger, but on an inaccurate or arbitrary symbolism.

Third-order emotions occur with the gradual abandonment of preconceptual levels and the development of the conceptual levels of cognition. In conjunction with the first- and second-order emotions, they offer the human being a very complicated and diversified emotional repertory. Language plays an important role in third-order emotions. The temporal representation is enlarged in the direction of both the past and the future. As an experiential phenomenon emotion has only one temporal dimension, which is the present. However, because of its cognitive components it is a present experience which may have a great deal to do with past experiences and with an envisioned future. A person may be happy or unhappy now because of what happened long ago or what he thinks may happen in the future.

Third-order emotions, although capable of

existing even before the occurrence of the conceptual level, expand and become much more complicated at the conceptual level. Important third-order emotions are sadness, hate, love, and joy. To discuss adequately what we know about them, which is little in comparison to what remains to be known, would fill many books. I shall take into consideration only one thirdorder emotion: sadness.

Sadness

Sadness is a specifically human phenomenon, although rudimentary forms of it or related emotions have been observed in other species of vertebrates. It may be referred to as a special pain which is not physical, but mental. The English word *pain* includes both physical and mental pain because they are similar as subjective experiences of suffering. If our general assumption about feeling is correct, sadness, like physical pain, must have been retained in evolution because it was useful for survival. It may have become a motivational force similar to other unpleasant feelings, whether sensations or emotions. The motivation would be an urge to remove the cause of the unpleasant feeling. This may seem hard to prove; take as examples seven situations in which a normal person is likely to feel sad or unhappy:

1. He hears the news that a person dear to him has suddenly died. He is in a state of grief and mourning.

2. A son or daughter has flunked an examination.

3. A sweetheart has openly and irrevocably declared that her love has come to an end.

4. He unexpectedly loses a position which has been held for many years with a feeling of commitment, loyalty, pleasure, and fulfillment.

5. He has been humiliated by his chief in the place of work.

6. He has been the victim of an injustice.

7. He recognizes that a basic position, a specific direction he has taken in life (for instance, allegiance to a cause, a person, a special type of work) is wrong. He has wasted time and energy, and must now change direction.

Our life experiences enable us to

understand how an individual who is faced with one or more of these seven circumstances may have emotions ranging from mild sadness to despondency, anguish, unhappiness, and severe sorrow.

An individual who expects an unhappy or dangerous event to happen is in a state of anxiety. But in the seven examples, the loss has already occurred or the damage has already taken place. Because the individual realizes that the damage has already taken place, he experiences not anxiety, but sadness.

It is evident that an appraisal of the situation has been a prerequisite for the sadness to occur. The individual not only realizes the impact of the undesirable event on his present life, but he is able to assess the negative effect that it will have on his future. To refer again to the seven examples, he no longer will enjoy the company of the deceased person; his son will not be promoted; he will no longer receive love from the sweetheart; he no longer will retain the coveted position; he has lost face or reputation among co-workers; he may not be able to undo the damage done to him, as people may really believe he is guilty; he has been a fool in devoting himself so much to an unworthy cause; and so on.

Some authors believe that feelings of sadness and depression are caused by a decrease of norepinephrine in certain parts of the central nervous system. It seems certain that a chemical change occurs in the brain of the individual who experiences sadness. But contrary to the position taken by Akiskal and McKinney (1975), it seems plausible that the leap is not from chemistry to psychology, but from psychology to chemistry. In other words, the cognitive appraisal of the event comes before the chemical change. If the chemical change is necessary for the subjective experience of sadness, then the chemical change must be responsible for another leap, from a chemical reaction to the psychological experience of sadness.

It is important to stress at this point how extensive the cognitive work is that prepares the ground for the feeling of sadness. To understand the meaning of the death of a person dear to us and the significance that his absence will have in our life, or to comprehend fully the meaning of a humiliation or a basic error that we have made, implies evaluating thousands of facts and their ramifications, myriads of ideas, and a plurality of feelings which are often discordant. First, billions of neurons do cognitive work in the neopallium; then sadness is experienced as the outcome of the cognitive work. The concerted functioning of all the neopallic neurons is transformed into an emotion, an experience of inner status.

In this book we shall not deal with the anatomical structures that mediate this transformation. From the classic work of Papez (1937) and those who have followed Papez's work, we know that a large number of neopallic structures must find pathways to some parts of the limbic system. But at this point already we can reflect upon a phenomenon which appears miraculous; that in as little time as a fraction of a second to a few seconds, the work of a multitude of neurons is transformed into an emotional experience. When we respond to a simple stimulus with an experience of inner status, the phenomenon may not appear impressive until we realize that the experience of inner status is the outcome of the concerted work of billions of neurons.

Similar phenomena, which include an enormous variation in the intensity or complexity of stimuli, occur throughout the nervous system. For instance, the auditory system can hear the weakest whisper and also hear and understand the meaning of an explosive sound, even though these two sound experiences vary as much as a trillionfold. The eyes can see visual images that vary a millionfold in their light intensities (Guyton, 1972). Thus some regions of the limbic system may also be capable of responding with a painful emotion to wave fronts of nervous stimulation varying enormously in size and coming from the neopallic areas.

It seems easy to establish that a cognitive work is necessary to experience normal sadness, just as we can ascertain easily that a change in the cognitive work may reverse the feeling of sadness. The following example will clarify this point. During the second World War some families were notified of a relative missing in action. The news generally provoked a great deal of sorrow and also anxiety, since the death of the missing person was not proved. When additional news arrived that confirmed the death of the soldier, any feeling of anxiety disappeared and only a profound feeling of sadness was experienced. In those rare instances, reported in the newspapers, in which the soldier who was thought to be dead was instead found to be alive and well, sadness immediately disappeared and was replaced by happiness and joy. It is thus clear that a change in the cognitive work can change the emotion. What remains to be demonstrated is how in the case of sadness the emotion becomes a motivational force.

Sadness—And Bereavement In Particular—As A Motivational Force

If sadness is like other unpleasant feelings, it must be a promoter of behavior which will lead to the disappearance of sadness. This function is easy to understand in the case of pain, hunger, thirst, tiredness, fear, and anxiety, which all lead to behavior that tends to avoid, remove, or prevent the cause of the feeling itself. But what can we do in the case of sadness, when the harmful event or the loss has already taken place? Moreover, when we feel sad we also feel less equipped to take any action whatsoever. In contrast to persons who are angry and ready to fight, or persons who are afraid and ready to flee, we feel slowed down in our activities and thought processes. In order to understand the phenomenon, we must consider some of the seven examples listed above. Let us consider in greater detail our first example of an individual who hears the news that a person he loves has unexpectedly died.

After he has understood and almost instantaneously evaluated what this death means to him, he experiences shock and then sadness; or to be exact, that particular type of normal sadness which is called bereavement, mourning, or grief. For a few days all thoughts connected with the deceased person bring about a painful, almost unbearable feeling. Any group of thoughts remotely connected with the dead person elicits sorrow. The individual cannot adjust to the idea that the loved person does not live any more. And since that person was so important to him, many of his thoughts or actions are directly or indirectly connected with the dead person and therefore elicit sad reactions. He finds himself searching for the dead person. When he sees a person who looks like the dead person, he has a fleeting impression, almost immediately corrected, that he sees the dead person. Nevertheless, after a certain period of time which varies from individual to individual, the person in mourning seems to become adjusted to the idea that the loved one is dead.

How is this change possible? If the individual is able to introspect, he will recognize that some clusters of thought have replaced the old ones which were connected with the departed. At first he had the impression at a conscious level that the painful thoughts about the departed person prevented him from thinking about anything else. But after some time he recognizes that the opposite is true: the painful thoughts attract new ones, as if they wanted to be replaced by new thoughts. This cognitive activity goes on until the grief work is completed.

At first there is an attempt to recapture the dead person, to make the deceased live again in dreams, daydreams, and fantasies. Because these attempts are doomed to fail, the individual is left with only one possibility, which is to rearrange the ideas that are connected with the departed. This rearrangement can be carried out in several ways, according to the person's mental predisposition. For example, he may come to consider the deceased no longer indispensable. He may associate the image of the dead person mainly with the qualities of that person which elicited pleasure, so that the image no longer brings mental pain but pleasure. Or he may think of the deceased's life as not really ended, but as being continued either in a different world or in this world through the lasting effects of the deceased's actions. Finally he may think that another person can replace the deceased one in his life; the deceased was not unique in every respect. Whatever the ideational rearrangement, there is no moving away from a physical source of discomfort as in pain, or from the source of danger as in fear. The moving away is only from certain chains of thought that perpetuate the feeling of sadness. It is not the passage of time that heals, but the rearrangement of ideas, which still may require a considerable amount of time.

As I wrote in *The Intrapsychic Self*,[10] sadness is an unpleasant emotion which has a tendency not to be extinguished rapidly, like rage, but to last. It does not have an impelling tendency toward immediate action and discharge, like rage and fear; it is neither centripetal, such as fear which is experienced as something directed from the frightening stimulus to the organism, nor centrifugal, such as rage which is experienced as being directed toward something outside of the organism. Although precipitated most of the time by certain events that occur in the external world, it is reflexive in the sense that it seems to reflect back to the organism that experiences it.

In summary, sadness slows our activities and lasts long enough in us not to evoke a prompt motor response. It favors slow mental processes which bring about a reorganization of thoughts about life directives, and eventually different purposeful behavior.

In children who are not mature enough to know that the loss is irreparable, the urge to recover the lost object is stronger than in adults, as Bowlby has described (1960a). Many authors (Anna Freud, 1960; Jacobson, 1971) doubt that the reaction of children to the loss of their mother can really be called mourning and not bereavement. At any rate, even if such a reaction is not equivalent to the mourning of adults, it is certainly a state of sadness following an unpleasant event.

Parkes (1964, 1965, 1972, 1973) has done the most extensive research on mourning. He described the effects of mourning or bereavement on sixty-six widows from several parts of England. He wrote that when a bereaved adult learns of the death of a loved person, he tends to call and search for that person. Since he knows, however, that the search is useless and painful, he denies the search. The result is a compromise, a partial expression of the search. Whereas the child cries and protests, as Bowlby described, the adult goes on searching. Parkes (1973) described a woman who was searching for her missing son. "She moves restlessly about the likely parts of the house scanning with her eyes and thinking of the boy; she hears a creak and immediately associates it with the sound of her son's footfall on the stair; she calls out, 'John, is that you?'"

In the process of searching there is in the beginning a motor hyperactivity which, according to Parkes, has the specific aim of finding the one who has died. This hyperactivity was already described by Lindemann: "The activity throughout the day of severely bereaved persons show remarkable changes. There is no retardation of action and speech; quite to the contrary, there is a rush of speed, especially when talking about the deceased. There is restlessness, inability to sit still, moving about in an aimless fashion, continually searching for something to do. There is, however, at the same time, a painful lack of capacity to initiate and maintain normal patterns of activity" (Lindemann, 1944). According to Parkes, after hyperactivity subsequent features are

preoccupation with the memory of the lost person, a scanning of perceptual stimulations to find evidence of the lost person, focusing attention on those parts of the environment that are associated with the deceased, and finally the conscious recognition of the urge to search for the lost person.

Parkes wrote that grief is commonly described as a process by which a person detaches himself from a lost object. Yet the bereaved person acts as if he wants restoration of the object. However, Parkes (1973) adds that "with repeated failure to achieve reunion, the intensity and duration of searching diminish, habituation takes place, the 'grief work' is done. It seems that the human adult has the same need to go through the painful business of pining and searching if he is to 'unlearn' his attachment to a lost person."

I believe that Parkes focuses on an early stage of mourning, after the period of initial shock and retardation. Parkes reaffirms what I have previously described (Arieti, 1959), that the bereaved individual becomes reactivated in the search of a restoration of the lost person. There is no longer retardation, but motor and mental hyperactivity which aims at retrieving the lost person. It seems to me that by enacting this unrealistic and futile search, the individual is behaving like a person who has undergone a trauma and dreams about it again and again in order to get used to the trauma, to become desensitized to it, or to diminish its emotional impact.

I disagree with Parkes that the "grief work" is done with the completion of the activities he described. If by grief work we mean reparative work, we must recognize that Parkes has described only the first part which is preparatory for the second.

With the first part of the grief work, the patient becomes partially desensitized to the loss but, having realized the futility of his efforts, he also becomes more open to realistic alternatives. He will accept the cognitive possibilities described: he no longer considers the deceased individual to be indispensable; he thinks the deceased is still alive through his works or in another world, or that the deceased can be replaced by another person; and so forth. The grief work is done and sadness disappears only when one or more of these alternatives are accepted and they elicit in the bereaved a different type of mental and motor behavior.

Alberta Szalita (1974) wrote about bereavement: "Whenever an individual suffers a loss . particularly a beloved person—he

normally undergoes a period of grief and mourning of varying intensity until he recovers the energy he invested in the lost object. The process of mourning is very painful. It is a travail that reconciles him to the loss and permits him to continue his life with unimpaired vigor, or even with increased vitality. A similar process takes place when one is confronted with a disappointment, failure, the loss of a love object through rejection, divorce, abandonment, and the like."

Szalita divides mourning into three stages: complete identification with the deceased, splitting of the identification, and a detailed review of the relationship. Szalita describes the third stage as "a somewhat detached appraisal of one's own conduct toward the lost object. The self-evaluation encompasses a painful working through of myriads of minute elements and a complete scanning of one's life. There can be no glossing over in this process; shallowness is incompatible with mourning. The result of 'digging in' is that one emerges as an integrated, enriched, and revitalized person." Szalita's third stage corresponds partially to the reparatory phase that I have described.

It is useful to stress again that the slowness produced by sadness has a purpose. In sadness, the reparatory work takes a long time. Quick actions are more difficult to implement, and so are propensities to make quick escapes in completely unrelated directions.

An additional aspect of the motivational meaning of mourning has been stressed by classic psychoanalysis since Freud wrote *Mourning and Melancholia* (1917). The bereaved person feels guilty for having survived the deceased person, for not having prevented his death, or more frequently for believing that he has wished his death. Such wishing may only have been unconscious, but the sadness is an expiation for guilt. Although it is true that these complexes can be traced in some people, especially in persons who become depressed to a pathological degree after the death of a close person (see chapter 6), it is very unlikely that this mechanism explains bereavement as a universal phenomenon.[11]

If we review the other six situations listed above in which a normal person is likely to feel sad or unhappy, the phenomenon of sadness will appear similar and yet in some respects simpler than bereavement.

First there is a cognitive appraisal of the event and its consequences, then a state of sadness and retardation, and finally the reparative work. The reparative work of sadness is generally more realistic and consists of less unrealistic fantasies, unless pathological complications ensue. For instance, the parent of the youngster who has flunked the examination will try to convince the child to study more intensely, try again, or change vocations. The person who has been abandoned by his sweetheart will reevaluate his love or try to find a new sweetheart. The person who recognizes that he is wrong in the special direction he has given to his life or in giving his allegiance to a wrong cause, person, or work generally does not respond with sadness to any specific event, but to a realization of the pattern of his life or to a new meaning that he gives to this pattern. This is actually one of the most frequent causes of sadness and depression, as we shall study in detail in chapter 6. The reappraisal of one's life may cause sorrow but if the sorrow work is successful, the individual may reacquire normality or at least avoid depression.

What we have illustrated so far seems to indicate beyond doubt that there is a purpose in sadness. Thus we can understand why evolution has selected sadness as one of the essential feelings in the gamut of human experience.

I am aware that this type of formulation may irritate those readers in scientific research who accept an exclusively deterministic explanation without the concept of purpose or selection. I wish to remind the reader that when in biological reports we use such expressions as "evolution has selected," we follow *une faison de parler*. We do not anthropomorphize a process which has taken millions of years to happen. We use human terms to refer to the fact that mutations not suitable to the survival of the species are more likely to disappear. The unfavorable mutations therefore are not reproduced, and only those that are statistically (even if not in individual cases) favorable to survival are perpetuated. Although in some specific states sadness may lead to depression and suicide, in the total picture of the human species it has positive survival value. Moreover, the feeling of sadness may deterministically be brought about by previous causes, but in the restricted human frame of reference it has a purpose and a beneficial effect for some members of our species. When we use psychodynamic concepts, we imply normal or abnormal purposes even if the whole process of life can be reinstated in the deterministic scheme of the cosmos (Arieti, 1967, 1970).

Other Aspects of Sadness

The purpose of sadness discussed in the previous section does not exclude the possibility that this feeling has other motivations and meanings.

For instance, some thinkers are inclined to see a certain appropriateness or correspondence between an adverse cognitive appraisal and sadness which is similar to the appropriateness between a positive appraisal and happiness.

What could be more appropriate than to feel sad when we learn that a friend has died or when we realize that our life has followed a wrong pattern? Would it not seem absurd to laugh in such circumstances? Thus should we not focus on the appropriateness of sadness in similar circumstances, rather than on its biological or psychodynamic function? Moreover, and notwithstanding what I have said earlier in this chapter, why should a symbolic value in sorrow and sadness not exist? Is not the unpleasantness of the sorrow a symbol (or partial reproduction) of the unpleasant event that caused it, just as joy and love are symbols of pleasant events?

On the other hand, the unpleasantness of an event may be a post hoc consideration. In other words, would we consider an event unfavorable or adverse if we did not experience sadness? Undoubtedly in a restricted human sense or at least in the adult human being, emotions can be evaluated in different ways. However, it seems almost evident in the case of sadness that the negative value of the experience appears to mirror the negative value of the event which caused it. In a certain way this appropriateness is inherent in the quality of the subjective experience, similar to what occurs in the experience of the baby who in its first day of life appreciates the negative value of pain.

Pleasantness and unpleasantness, appropriateness and inappropriateness, again may be the result of associations between stimuli and responses which have been retained because they are favorable to survival. For instance, we know of nothing that seems more favorable to procreation than to associate reproductive activities with the pleasure of sex. In other cases associations between cognitive events and emotional responses or somatic concomitants of these emotions remain obscure: we do not know why we blush when we are embarrassed, yawn when we are bored, and laugh when we hear a funny story.

Transformation of Sadness

In many cases the psyche does not tolerate more than a certain amount of sadness. These are situations in which some individuals seem to function more favorably or less unfavorably under the influence of other feelings, even if those feelings are also negative in value. Sadness thus is transformed into anxiety, rage, anger, and hypochondriacal or psychosomatic mechanisms.

These outcomes will be illustrated in other chapters.

An important mechanism in the transformation of sadness has been used throughout the history of mankind, but it is available only to a few people. It consists of the attempt to project the state of sorrow into the external world and to believe it is in the external world that the sorrow work has to be done. At times the imperfection of human nature, society, history, or fate is seen as the object of sorrow. At other times it is the burden that society, religion, or our consciences compel us to bear. In other words, the sadness of the individual becomes enlarged or rationalized as a pessimistic philosophy of life, epistemology, and cosmology. Such a philosophy can always be justified, since as we can always find undesirable aspects in the world. The individual generally concludes that he must accept the ineluctably unhappy state of the world. He sees his own personal unhappiness as part of the total picture and therefore more tolerable.

Some great thinkers have been able to influence society and culture with this point of view. In its turn, culture has become pessimistic and melancholy and has facilitated a state of sadness or melancholia in society at large. Thus a vicious circle ensues and a tradition of social melancholia becomes established. This matter will be discussed in greater detail in chapter 16.

Unresolved Sadness and Depression

In some cases of psychiatric relevance the state of sadness is not resolved and becomes transformed into a more intense unhappy feeling called depression. This feeling often replaces all other feelings except those, like guilt and selfdepreciation, which are associated with sorrow. In some cases anxiety remains for a long time, but eventually anxiety is also submerged by the overall feeling of depression. Any thought is negative and reinforces the depression. Thus thoughts become slow and less frequent, perhaps in an attempt to reduce the quantity of suffering that they cause. If painful thoughts could be eliminated, there would be no depression; but these thoughts are never eliminated. In some situations, as in reactive depression, painful thoughts for the most part remain conscious. In other conditions the thoughts or systems of thought which cause the depression become unconscious or submerged by a general feeling of depression. Consequently the patient is not able to say why he is depressed.

I have suggested that intense depression has (among others) the same function as repression in other psychiatric conditions. Perhaps it is a special type of repression; the cognitive part is repressed, but the painful feeling is experienced at the level of consciousness.

I am aware, however, of another frequent mechanism in people who have experienced depression in the past. They repress painful ideas in order to avert the depression. The attempt is unsuccessful; the ideas, although unconscious, continue to cause conscious depression. Some patients express themselves in this or a similar way: "I woke up this morning, and I was immediately hit by an intense feeling of depression. I don't know where it came from." Other patients attribute their depression to unhappy ideas that they have about themselves, the future, or life—the triad that Beck has described so well. What Beck does not indicate is that patients use these thoughts to justify their depression. Beck is correct to the extent that these thoughts reinforce the depression which comes from other sources. They add a secondary depression to the original, and only important, one.

In more serious cases, thinking is reduced to a minimum and retardation becomes more pronounced even to the degree of stupor. In these circumstances the retardation of mental processes becomes a self-defeating mechanism. Cognitive elements are very rare or disappear completely and the intense, agonizing feeling of depression remains almost as sole possessor of the psyche. The suffering is so intense that when a patient becomes slightly less depressed and more capable of thinking and moving, he starts to conceive suicidal plans in order to put an end to his suffering.

At this point what is perhaps the most crucial question in this book must be asked: Why do sadness or sorrow work fail in some individuals and depression ensue? At the present stage of our knowledge, no hypothesis can be verified by acceptable scientific standards. We shall examine several possibilities.

1. The biologically oriented psychiatrist is inclined to think that a faulty biochemical process is responsible.

For instance, catecholamines are not being produced in a quantity sufficient to restore the organism after the psychological event of sadness has depleted the brain's biogenic amines.

2. The neurologically inclined psychiatrist can think that the part of the limbic brain that receives the stimulation from pathways coming from the neopallic cognitive areas is particularly sensitive and responds excessively. It could also be that, for reasons so far unknown, different parts of the brain are stimulated concertedly, involving unusual neuronal pathways which lead to depression. Unfortunately this hypothesis has not received the consideration that it deserves, presumably because it is very difficult to investigate experimentally. Incidentally, this hypothesis does not exclude an altered biochemical mechanism. The neurological alteration may lead to a biochemical disorder.

3. The reparative process (sorrow work) cannot take place because the person is not psychologically equipped for it. Life circumstances,

as well as psychological patterns followed by the patient, have not prepared him for the sorrow work. He has no choice; he is not able to solve psychologically his sorrow or

sadness, and pathological depression results.

A psychodynamic approach to depression studies this third possibility. Incidentally, this possibility does not exclude that some biological variables may make the psychological repair work more difficult. In these cases a combination of psychological and neurochemical factors are the determinants of the depression.

A frequent criticism of the psychodynamic explanation for depression is that there is no failure of the sorrow work, no preceding sadness. Many patients have become depressed immediately, without any antecedent and external precipitating factor. If this is the case, we have to attribute the phenomenon exclusively to a faulty neurological or biochemical endogenous mechanism.

In my experience, patients whose depressions do not seem to be precipitated by psychological factors have been unaware of these factors. They have followed life patterns, sustained by cognitive components whose depressogenic value was kept in a state of unconsciousness or dim consciousness. Moreover, these rigid and static life patterns have prevented any alternative directions and any reparative work. The study of these life patterns constitutes the major part of the psychodynamic approach of this book.

It is true that many depressed patients— and, incidentally, many people who experience normal sorrow—can be relieved with ingestion of certain drugs. This possibility does not disprove the psychological origin of the feeling. It proves only that whatever physiological or biochemical intermediary exists between the psychological factors and the subjective experience can be altered. Exclusive concern with the biochemical intermediary stage is a reductionist approach. Nature has equipped us to respond to adverse aspects of life not only with biological changes but also with our sorrow —that is, with psychological participation. When sorrow is not solved and depression ensues, we must help the person to acquire a different pattern of psychological participation.

Notes

[9] In an article published in 1960 I described sensations and emotions as experiences of inner status, or subjective conditions of the organism. In my book *The Intrapsychic Self* (1967) I also examined in detail the main emotions. In this section I discuss this topic briefly and only in relation to the main theme of the book.

[10] In that book I called sadness "normal depression," a term I no longer use.

[11] For additional studies on bereavement, the reader is referred to Parkes (1972), and Schoenberg et al. (1975).

PSYCHODYNAMICS OF SEVERE DEPRESSION

Silvano Arieti

In the previous chapter we have seen that an unsolved state of sorrow tends to develop into a state of depression. Because they are most suitable to didactical examination, we predominantly have taken into consideration states of sorrow that unfold rather quickly as the result of specific, mostly sudden events. In practice we find that many states of sadness leading to severe depression have a long course, either chronic or subchronic, liminal or subliminal. We also find that in many cases in which a specific occurrence was the obvious and major precipitating factor, a subliminal state of sadness resulting from previous contingencies preexisted. Thus it is important to study the longitudinal psychodynamic history of each patient.

A psychodynamic history is not just a sequence of events from birth to the present time, but an unfolding of psychological forces which derive from the interplay between external and internal events.

As mentioned in chapter 1, every human being is in a fundamental state of receptivity; that is, ready and capable of being influenced by the environment. But human beings are not to be defined only in terms of this state of receptivity. Every human being even in early childhood has another basic function which is integrative activity (Arieti, 1977). Just as the transactions with the world not only inform but transform the individual, the individual transforms these transactions with his integrative activity and in turn he is informed and transformed by these transformations. No influence is received like a direct and immutable message. Multiple

processes involving interpersonal and intrapsychic dimensions go back and forth.

The object of this chapter is to describe the way the environment influences the future severely depressed patient and the way he integrates these influences. It will become apparent that these ways are quite different from those of the normal person or the typical schizophrenic patient.

Childhood

As a rule, the childhood of a person who as an adult suffers from a form of severe depression has not been so traumatic as the childhoods of people who become schizophrenic or even seriously neurotic.

The parents of the patient generally give a picture of cohesiveness and stability. Only in a minority of cases is there serious talk of divorce. The family gives the appearance of having stable foundations and adhering to the conventions of society. The family conflicts, schisms, and special constellations described for families of schizophrenics are not seen as frequently in the families of patients suffering from affective disorders. When they exist, they are less pronounced than in the families of schizophrenics.

The future severely depressed patient generally is born in a home which is willing to accept him and to care for him. The word accept has a special meaning in this context; the mother is duty-bound and willing to administer to the baby as much care as he requires, and she is willing to provide everything for him that he needs. This willingness of the mother is in turn accepted by the child, who is willing to accept everything he is offered; that is, early in life the child is very receptive to the influence (or giving) of the significant adult (parent). There are no manifestations of resistance toward accepting this influence, such as autistic manifestations or attempts to prevent or retard socialization that one finds in schizophrenia (Arieti, 1974). If we use Martin Buber's terminology (1937), we may say that the "Thou" or the other is immediately accepted and introjected. The "Thou" is at first the mother, but this receptivity to the mother enhances a receptivity for both parents and all other important surrounding adults, and promotes a willingness to accept them with their symbols and values. It also promotes a certain readiness to accept their food (either the milk of the mother or regular food) and thus predisposes some people (but by no means all) to overeating, obesity, and the seeking of compensation from food when other satisfactions are not available.

This receptivity to others and willingness to introject the favors of others at this early age promotes special personality traits in the future patient. He tends to become an extrovert and also a conformist, willing to accept what he is given by his surroundings not only in material things, but also in terms of habits and values, and to rely less than the average person on his autonomous resources. This readiness to accept —this psychological receptivity—will predispose him also to pathological or exaggerated introjection; that is, he tends to depend excessively on others for certain aspects of life which will be considered later.

In the second year of life (or earlier, according to some authors) a new attitude on the part of the mother drastically changes the environment in which the child is growing. At times the sudden change is experienced as a severe trauma. The mother continues to take care of the child but considerably less so than before, and now she makes many demands on him. The child receives care and affection provided that he accepts the expectations his parents have for him and he tries to live up to them.

This brusque change in the parents' attitude is generally the result of many factors. Predominantly, their attitude toward life in general tends to evoke in the child an early sense of duty and responsibility: what is to be obtained must be deserved. The parents are generally dissatisfied with their own lives and at times harbor resentment toward the children who represent increased work and responsibility. However, this hostility is seldom manifested openly; it generally is manifested by the fact that the parents overly increase their expectations.

Thus the child finds his environment changed from one which predisposed him to great receptivity, to one of great expectation. These dissimilar environments actually are determined by a common factor; the strong sense of duty that compelled the mother to do so much for her baby is now transmitted at an early age to the child himself. Frequently in families of depressed patients there are many children. When the future patient is in his second year of life, a sibling often is already born and the mother lavishes her care on the newborn with the same duty-bound generosity that she previously had for the patient. This of course makes the change in the environment more marked for the patient.

This displacement by a younger sibling seems to be important in the dynamics of many cases of manic-depressive psychosis and other forms of severe depression, although no statistical proof of it can be given. Statistical studies so far have concerned themselves more with the order of birth (that is, whether the patient is the first-born child, second-born, etc.).

[12]

In many cases the brusque change had to occur because of unexpected events: the child had to be abandoned by the mother because of illness, economic setback, forced emigration, or political persecution. The child then was left in the custody of an aunt, grandmother, cousin, stranger, or orphan asylum and was subjected to a violent and unmitigated experience of loss.

For some patients the abrupt change that we have described has already taken place at the time of weaning. Future affective patients are generally breast-fed in their infancy and then suddenly deprived of mother's milk. No bottles, rubber nipples, or pacifiers are used. There is a sharp transition from the breast to the glass. In a minority of patients this loss of the breast plays an important role.

In many other patients the abrupt change occurs later, generally in the preschool years but at times even in grammar-school years. (See the case of Mrs. Fullman in chapter 10.) In other cases specific events take place which make the child feel threatened in his main love relationship. The change may be in the composition of the family, in the attitude of the parents, or on account of some unusual event. When the patient gives to the therapist an account of this change as he remembers it much later, the threat seems in some cases at least to have been experienced in an exaggerated manner. However, in many other cases there seems to have been a justification for an intensely unpleasant feeling. In still other cases the child does not remember the experience of having been threatened, but he remembers acting as if he had been threatened, and indeed at times he remembers facts which should have threatened him. The word threat and not loss is used here, although the child in many instances has sustained a loss (of mother, maternal maid, love, etc.). If the child experiences the disturbing event as a loss, he tends to become immediately depressed. But the person who becomes depressed only in adult life, somehow in childhood was able to compensate partially for this traumatic experience, or to experience it as a threat for which he had to find coping devices.

Freud (1917) suggested that the withdrawal

of love, approval, and support on the part of the parent or parent surrogate during an important stage of development predisposes a person to depression in life. Abraham (1916) felt that depression occurring later in life was predisposed by a withdrawal of love in very early childhood and fixation at the oral stage. No matter how devastating these events have been in some cases, patients who become depressed only in adult life have had throughout their childhood a capacity to muster defenses which somewhat diminished the sense of loss. The loss was transformed into a threat with which the child had to learn to deal. Some stability and feeling of hope was maintained.

How does the child try to adjust to the new threatening situation? The child who later is likely to develop an affective disorder tends to adopt special mechanisms. A common one (although as we shall see later, it is decreasing in frequency) is to find security by accepting parental expectations no matter how onerous they are. The child does not reject the parents emotionally, or avoid them as the schizoid often does, but he consciously accepts them. He must live up to their expectations no matter how heavy the burden. It is only by complying, obeying, and working hard that he will recapture the love or state of bliss which he used to have as a baby; or at the very least he will maintain that moderate love which he is receiving now. Love is still available, but not as a steady flow. The flow is intermittent and conditioned, and therefore it does not confer security. The child feels that he will be punished if he does not do what he is supposed to, and mother may withdraw her love totally. At the same time that the anxiety of losing the mother's love occurs, the child is given hope that he will be able to retain this love or recapture it if and when it is lost. The child thus feels he has a choice, or the freedom, to retain the parental love. No matter what he chooses, however, he has a hard price to pay: submission or rejection. He also feels that mother is not bad in spite of her appearance; on the contrary, she is good. She is good even in punishing him, because by punishing him she wants to redeem him, make him worthy again of her love. Thus the mechanism is different from what occurs in many preschizophrenics; although the future affective patient has an image of himself as being bad, he does not feel that he is beyond the possibility of redemption as the preschizophrenic often does. The anxiety about being unable to fulfill parental expectations changes into guilt feelings. If affection or forgiveness is not forthcoming, the child feels that it is his own fault; he has not lived up to what was expected of him, and he feels guilty. When he feels guilty he again expects punishment. He wants to be punished because punishment is the lesser of the evils; he would rather be punished than lose his mother's love. If he is not punished, he often works harder in order to punish himself.

A little later, but at a very early age, many of these children assume responsibilities such as the support of the family. If they engage in a career, it is often in order to bring honor and prestige to the family. In a certain number of cases, the family belongs to a marginal group of society because of religious or ethnic minority status or other reasons, and the child feels that it is his duty to rescue the family with his own achievement. In all these cases we can recognize a pattern of compliance, submission, and selfimposed hard discipline.

In some patients incestuous wishes toward parents and, as frequently, toward siblings of the opposite sex further elicit strong guilt feelings for which the patient feels he must atone by making even more rigid the pattern of relating that we have described.

Other findings make the picture more complicated and difficult to understand. For instance, the parents of some patients appear to be not strict, but overindulgent. This is possible because in this second stage of childhood the parents do not need to enforce any rules with their actions. The rules, the principles, have already been incorporated by the child. As a matter of fact, some of the parents now regret that the children take rules with such seriousness.

Before proceeding to describe other possibilities in the early family life of the depressed adult, we must make some theoretical considerations which take as a paradigm the situation of compliance and submission that we have described. (We shall analyze variants later.) This interpersonal relation based on compliance and placation has predisposed the child to select and adopt specific ways of facing the world, others, and himself. We do not refer exclusively or predominantly to enduring patterns of behavior, but to ways of thinking and choosing that are related to the integrative activity of the child. At times this integrative activity remains only a predisposition to live according to some schemata. At other times the integrative activity leads to the organization of patterns as rigid as imprintings which last the whole life, especially if they are reinforced by repetition of the same events. These patterns of living do not consist only of movements, or of specific external behaviors. They are cognitive-affective structures which have been built as a result of learning, in the act of facing the early interpersonal situation. To be specific, they are built on the appraisal of external events, the ability to choose some actions instead of others, and the capacity to anticipate the effect that these actions will have on the interpersonal environment.

A theory based on the prevalence of certain cognitive constructs is at variance with psychological and psychiatric conceptions that exclusively see patterns of living as reactions to environmental situations. The concept of reaction which is derived from a behavioristic frame of reference implies almost total passivity in regard to the influence of the environment, and deterministic ineluctability. According to the interpretation offered in this book, the patient sizes up a particular environment and relates to it in the best possible way or, rather, interrelates in the roles of both subject and object. The cognitive construct which receives our major consideration in this book has to do with a person who is very important to the individual in question. I have called this person the *significant other*. The significant other, generally the mother, is the adult from whom the child expects nourishment, acceptance, recognition, love, and respect.

In the interpersonal relation that we have described, the child develops an attitude of excessive compliance in dealing with the significant other. Each individual relates to more than one person and also to groups; for instance, to the family in its totality. Nevertheless, I have referred to the significant other in the singular because at this stage of development the dyadic relation is by far the prevailing one. The interpersonal pattern of behavior that the child displays in relation to the mother and which he later generalizes to his dealings with other people can be seen to derive from the interpersonal branch of the basic construct that we are considering. However, the original construct has another branch, the intrapersonal, which is expanding rapidly. It has to do mainly with the child's self-image; how the child sees himself in consequence of the way he believes other people think of him, and the way he evaluates himself as a consequence of the way he deals with people.

Each important construct can be seen as having a psychological bifurcation, with one intrapersonal branch and the other interpersonal. Both branches are intrapsychic— even the interpersonal one. They are internal structures that lead to certain external behavior and inner elaboration of this behavior. In the construct based on the relation of excessive receptivity and compliance that we have described, we can recognize a structure, a choice, a purpose—the realization of loss or threat and the attempt to cope with it.

We will now describe other situations and inner constructs and show how they predispose the patient to consequent patterns that make it difficult for him to do sorrow work, and thus make him likely to become depressed sometime in his adult life. In many instances we find that as a child the patient believed that he could reacquire love, approval, and consideration not just by complying, obeying, and working hard, but by converging all or almost all of his efforts toward a goal—for instance, toward becoming an outstanding man, a leader, an actor, or a great lover. In late childhood and early adolescence these aims were fantasized in terms of becoming a great scientist, writer, industrialist, winner of the Nobel prize, and so forth. In other cases the aim was to find a great love or a mission. Although early in life this pattern was developed in order to please or placate the significant other, it soon became an aim in itself. The significant other lost significance and was replaced gradually by a significant goal. The patient came to live for that goal exclusively. His whole selfesteem and reason for living were based on reaching the goal.

To have goals and life aspirations is a common occurrence in normal children and adolescents. As a matter of fact, it is a desirable trait for the young individual to conceive of some directions for his life and even to have fantasies and daydreams about them. However, in the person who later becomes seriously depressed, the significant goal occupies the major part of the psyche and leaves no room for other goals, or for flexibility toward other possibilities. Unless the trend is later corrected, these children become not only achievement-oriented to the exclusion of other aspects of life, but oriented toward achieving only in a given way.

Unless they shift their orientation—and fortunately many of them do —already at a young age they appear self-centered and selfish, at times even oblivious of the needs and feelings of others, including those close to them. Whereas the individual who is concerned with pleasing the significant other maintains an important interpersonal relation, even one of dubious value, the person who lives for the significant goal tends to be aloof and self-involved.

A third important pattern with which the child tries to cope with the sudden change in environmental circumstances is the attempt to make himself more babyish, more in need of the significant other. He develops a pattern of dependency. If the child makes himself aggressively dependent, the mother or other important adults are forced to reestablish an atmosphere of babyhood or young childhood, that is, of early bliss. The child and later the adult will develop a very demanding and at the same time clinging, dependent type of personality.

Since the 1950s this last pattern of living has become much more common at least in the United States. The increased frequency may be related to different fashions of raising children. The child senses permissiveness in the family environment and believes that by making claims and being demanding, he will reestablish the previous position of blissful dependency.

We must clarify the fact that in spite of these predominant patterns being established in childhood, secondary patterns coexist in all patients who later develop an affective disorder. The child develops a strong resentment toward the significant other who in the first type of mechanism imposes so much, or who in the third type does not give enough. Such resentment manifests itself in attacks of rage, anger, rebellion, or even violence. When such anger becomes manifest, it is often enough to dispel an oncoming feeling of sadness. For this reason, some therapists believe that any depression hides an underlying anger. This is true only to a limited extent: the anger is consequent to a situation which already existed and was unacceptable to the child. Anger alone is not a solution to the conflict-laden situation, although it may be a temporary defense against depression.

Feelings of anger in many cases are promptly checked and repressed, not only in childhood but throughout the life of the patient. Sadistic thoughts and impulses are at times very pronounced but seldom acted out. Consequent guilt feelings are brought about by these impulses, as well as feelings of unworthiness. The patient soon learns that rebellion does not pay: on the contrary, it increases the atonement he must undergo later. The stronger his sadistic impulses, the stronger the masochistic tendencies become. He soon desires peace at any cost, so that any compromise is worthy of peace. The mechanism which permits him to maintain a certain equilibrium is the repression of this resentment. However, the resentment is retained unconsciously, and it appears in dreams and occasional outbursts which do reach consciousness. In children and adolescents who have adopted the second pattern, there are also episodes of anger and rebellion. They do not want to sacrifice everything for the sake of the significant goal. They go on sprees of indolence, effervescence, or erratic behavior. These sprees, however, remain eposodic and do not become prominent features.

There is an additional dynamic mechanism which is found in some cases of manicdepressive psychosis. The child senses that the acceptance or introjection of parents is too much of a burden and, without realizing it, shifts the direction of his incorporations to other adults in the environment (much older siblings, uncles, aunts, grandparents, friends, etc.) whom he internalizes instead of parents. Not only does the common tendency of children to introject adults become exaggerated, but peripheral adults become parentlike figures. The child unconsciously resorts to this mechanism in order to decrease the burden of the parental introjection, but in many cases this defense does not prove useful. As Fromm-Reichmann (1949) remarked, there will be no single significant adult to whom the patient can relate in a meaningful way. The relationship with these other grownups is again determined by a utilitarian purpose, duty, or role. The introjection of such adults eventually fails to provide what the child needs and may end by confusing him (how can he satisfy all the adults?) and increasing his burden and feeling of guilt.

The personality of the patient who develops an affective disorder is partially determined by one of the three main inner constructs and related patterns of living described in the previous section, and also by what has been accrued or brought about with these patterns. Even after a pattern has become prevalent, the individual is capable of dealing with the environment in a relatively large variety of ways. However, a certain rigidity of personality can be detected, and his future actions are more easily predicted. Finally the prevailing pattern becomes almost exclusively used.

First I will describe the personality of patients who have tried to adapt to their initial traumatic environment by adopting a pattern of placation. The first question which comes to mind is whether this type of personality corresponds to types already described in the psychiatric literature— for instance, to the compliant or moving-toward-people personality described by Karen Homey (1945, 1950).

This type of personality certainly has some characteristics in common with Horney's compliant personality, and perhaps it is a special variety of it. However, it has some characteristics of its own. Horney's compliant person manifests this attitude toward life in general and in many interpersonal exchanges, but the future severely depressed patient is more restrictive or discriminating. His placating attitude is manifested not toward life in general, but exclusively or at least in much more accentuated forms toward a person, the parents, or an institution. He generally converges the majority of his dealings on a person or institution. However, if we take into consideration a large number of these people, we find in them strong feelings of patriotism, religiosity, and loyalty to a political party or to their family. These people often wish to have a military or an ecclesiastic career. These institutions and organizations are unconsciously or subconsciously experienced as parents to be placated.

Group loyalty and *esprit de corps* play an important part in the psychological constellation of this personality type. Under the pretense of belonging to a group, a close-knit family, or an organization, the individual hides his loneliness.

In many cases we find a self-conscious individual, always motivated by duty, with the type of personality Riesman et al. (1950) called inner-directed. Often this devotion to duty assumes the form of devotion to order. Abraham (1924) described the rigid need for order, cleanliness, and stubbornness of the predepressed person. He mentions also his perseverence and solidity.

Shimoda (1961), a Japanese author who has studied depression deeply, refers to the tendency of the predepressed to certain thoughts and feelings. These persons appear to Shimoda to have integrity and to inspire a feeling of reliance.

Tellenbach (1974), a German author who has studied melancholia from different angles, also describes how the predepressed person craves order, cleanliness, and regularity. He expects a great deal from himself and tries to do even more. Tellenbach reports accurate clinical descriptions of patients who throughout their lives were ruled by this need to search for order and regularity, and to work as much as possible. Tellenbach does not try to explain, however, how this tendency originated.

According to my own experience, this type of predepressed person occasionally succeeds in overcoming some of his difficulties. He may even be able to channel them in original ways and become creative in special fields; but if he does not overcome his difficulties and spends all his energies to placate others, he does not unfold his creative possibilities and remains an imitator. However, what he tries to do, he does well. He has deep convictions and his life is motivated by principles. He must be a dedicated person. He is generally efficient and people who do not know him well have the impression that he is a welladjusted, untroubled individual.

On the contrary, he is not a happy man.[13] He selects a mate not because he loves her, but because she "needs" him. He will never divorce the mate because she is in terrible need of him. At the same time he blames himself for being so egotistical as to think that he is indispensable. The necessity to please others and to act in accordance with their expectations, or in accordance with the principles that he has accepted, makes him unable to get really in touch with himself. He does not listen to his own wishes; he does not know what it means to be himself. He works incessantly and yet has feelings of futility and emptiness. At times he conceals his unhappiness by considering what he has accomplished, just as he conceals his loneliness by thinking of the group to which he belongs. But when he allows himself to experience these feelings of unhappiness, futility, and unfulfillment, he misinterprets them again. He tends to believe that he is to be blamed for them. If he is unhappy or finds no purpose in life, it must be his fault, or he must not be worthy of anything else. A vicious circle is established which repeats itself and increases in intensity, often throughout the life of the patient, unless fortunate circumstances or psychotherapy intervene. Thus the inner construct that was described in the previous section becomes more entrenched and more and more acquires the originally conceptualized feelings of duty and guilt.

The patient often has partial insight into his own mechanisms but he does not know how to solve them. For instance, he is willing to accept the role in the family and in society which has been assigned to him, and yet later he scolds himself for playing this role, for not being spontaneous. But if he tries to refuse the role, he has guilt feelings. His conclusion is that no matter how he tries to solve his problems, he will feel he has made the wrong choice. A patient told me that she "felt like a little girl who pretends to be grown-up but is not. I am acting." But she must live in that way; that was her duty. It was her fault that she "acted" and did not accept social behavior as being spontaneous or real-life.

The patient also tends to put his superiors or teachers in a parental, authoritarian role. Quite often he feels angry at them as they seem to expect too much, or because they themselves have been found to be at fault. The patient does not know how to act: Should he continue to accept the authority of these people and the burden that acceptance implies, or should he remove them from the pedestal? But if he removes them, there will be a void. His authorities are part of him, his values, and the symbolic world upon which he sustains himself, and to do without them is impossible. Furthermore, he would feel very guilty. The patient often realizes (as Cohen and his co workers illustrated, 1954) that he tends to underestimate himself. It is his duty to undersell himself. On the other hand, he tends to blame himself for underestimating himself and giving himself no chance to develop his own talents and potential abilities. The patient is becoming more rigid: what used to be a defense, or a practical way to get along sufficiently well with people in everyday living, becomes a character armor. At times the rigidity of thinking and acting slips into obsessive-compulsive symptoms. Some patients are often diagnosed, with with some justification, as obsessive-compulsive.

In spite of the characteristics so far described, in many cases the patient succeeds in giving the impression that he is able to live independently or be really involved in his work. In many cases, however, he eventually becomes anchored to a person whom he needs to please, follow, and receive approval from. At this point we recognize that the equilibrium he has been able to maintain is precarious and sustained mainly or exclusively in relation to the person whom he must please. This person is no longer the significant other; at this point he is what I have called the *dominant other* (Arieti, 1962). The relation between the patient and the dominant other is not just one of submission on the part of the patient and domination on the part of the other.

With this attitude are feelings of affection, attachment, love, friendship, respect, and dependency, so that the relationship is a very complicated one. The dominant other is experienced by the patient not only as a person who demands a great deal, but also as a person who gives a great deal. And as a matter of fact, he either does give a great deal or is put by the patient into a giving role. The patient can no longer accept himself unless the dominant other accepts him, and he is unable to praise himself unless the dominant other praises him or is interpreted by the patient as praising him. As Bemporad wrote (1970), the patient is incapable of autonomous gratification. The fundamental characteristics in the relationship are the inequality in the two roles and the fact that the patient is so anchored to the dominant other that he cannot establish a deep or complete relation to any other person. Although this state of affairs was tolerable when the significant other was the mother and the patient was the child, it is no longer so and becomes maladaptive. The same construct that was applied to the childhood situation is used, and in some respects it has become more inflexible than it was then.

The dominant other provides the patient with the evidence, either real or illusory—or at least the hope—that acceptance, love, respect, and recognition of his human worth and meaning of his life are acknowledged by at least one other person. The dominant other is represented most often by the spouse. In the predominantly patriarchal structure of our society the dominant other is often the male and the submissive partner is the female. We shall return to this aspect of the problem in greater detail later.

Far less often in the role of the dominant other are, in order of frequency, the mother, a person to whom the patient was romantically attached, an adult child, a sister, the father. The dominant other also frequently is represented, through anthropopathy, by the firm where the patient works or a social institution to which he belongs such as the church, a political party, the army, a club, and so forth. All these dominant others are symbolic of the depriving mother, or to be more accurate, of the once-giving and later depriving mother. If the real mother is still living and is the dominant other, she acts in two ways; her role is actual in the present and also symbolic of her old role. If the dominant other dies, he becomes even more powerful through the meanings attached to his death.

The second type of predepressed person, who is characterized by the pursuit of a significant goal, gradually becomes haunted by a dominant goal. The dominant goal is omnipresent, always lurking about; it determines most actions of the patient and excludes many others. The goal as a rule is grandiose, like winning the Nobel prize or becoming the chief of the firm, and the actions of the patient can be interpreted as being motivated by the attempt to attain what his grandiose self-image demands. However, I do not believe that the dominant goal is exactly the same as the grandiose image described by Karen Homey (1945). Again, perhaps it is a variety of her concept, the variety which occurs in people prone to develop a severe depression.

The dominant goal is conscious, although the patient is not aware of the magnitude of its role and all its ramifications. The dominant goal seems more plausible and more realistic than Horney's idealized image: some people do reach their dominant goal. The patient certainly works hard and does his best to reach it. Although he is a daydreamer, his investment in achievement is used not only in daydreaming, but in acting as efficiently as he can. He does not postpone. The attainment of the dominant goal seems to be motivated by a thirst for glory. In most cases, however, it is more than that; it is a search for love. Unconsciously the patient feels that he will be worthy of love from others or from himself only if he succeeds in achieving the dominant goal. Often at a conscious level too, the search for the dominant goal coincides with the search for a perfect love.

Not so subtle as in the other types of predepressed personality is a relationship of dependency in which the mechanism of obviously leaning on mother and maternal substitutes has been adopted after the initial trauma in childhood. Contrary to the types previously described, this third type includes people who even at a superficial examination appear maladjusted. These patients have never forgotten the bliss of their first year of life and still expect or demand a continuation of it. They demand and expect gratification from others, and feel deprived and sad when they do not get what they expect. They are demanding but not aggressive in the usual sense of the word, because they do not try to get what they want through their own efforts: they expect it from others. They have not developed that complex of duty and hard work typical of the complying, introjecting patient.

These patients alternate between feeling guilty and having the desire to make other people feel guilty. They generally find one person on whom to depend, and they make this other person feel guilty if he does not do what they want. The sustaining person (generally the spouse) is empowered with the capacity to make the patient happy or unhappy and is supposed to be responsible for the patient's despair and helplessness. He also plays a dominant role in the life of the patient, but only because the patient expects a great deal from him, not because he makes demands on the patient. Relatively often in this group we find women who depend entirely on their husbands, who are generally much older. In these cases the dominant other is not only the person who is supposed to accept, love, respect the patient, but also the person who protects and gives material things. At times the request is immense: the patient almost seems to request, metaphorically, milk or blood.

In some cases there is an apparent variation in the picture when the patient tries desperately to submerge himself in work and activities, hoping that eventually he will find something to do which will make him worthy of recognition from other people. Whereas the first two types of predepressed persons looked inward for a solution to their conflicts, the third type looks externally for the solution.

A fourth type is observed in some patients who develop manic-depressive psychosis. It is manifested either as the prevailing type of personality or as a temporary characterological structure which from time to time replaces one of the three pictures previously described. This fourth type, the forerunner of the manic, is lively, active, hearty, and friendly. On closer scrutiny the person's apparent health and liveliness are found to be superficial. In a certain way the patient actually escapes into actions or reality, but he remains shallow and dissatisfied. If he happens to be engaged in work in which action is required rather than concentration, he may do well and maintain a satisfactory level of adjustment; otherwise he may sooner or later get into trouble. He claims that he has many friends and the interpersonal relations seem warm and sincere, but they are superficial and lack real kinship. One patient said, "I joke, I laugh, I pretend; I appear radiant and alive, but deep down I am lonely and empty." This type of person is only in certain respects the opposite of the duty-bound individual. He tries to escape from his inner-directedness, but he does not correspond to what Riesman called the "other directed" person. Imitating Riesman's terminology, we could call this hypomaniclike person outer-directed but not other-directed. He does not escape into others; he escapes from his inner self, because the inner self has incorporated the burdening others. He escapes into the world of superficial reality where meditations, reflections, or deep emotions are unnecessary. His main attitude can be interpreted as a great denial of everything which, if admitted, could lead to depression.

Such an individual may at times seem so free as to be considered psychopathic. Actually, it is his deep concern with conventional morality that often leads to this pseudopsychopathic escape. Some of the pseudo-psychopathic hypomanics have demonstrated asocial behavior since childhood when, for example, in order to escape from inner and external restrictions, they ran away from home or school.

These affective, prepsychotic personality types are seldom seen in pure culture. When the patient changes or alternates from one of the first three types of personality to the fourth, he presents the so-called cyclothymic personality.

The Development of the Severe Attack

The types of personality described in the previous section lead not to a stable equilibrium, but to an almost constant state of dissatisfaction and sadness (or, in some cases, hypomanic denial of sadness). If we closely examine the period of time that precedes the depression— and this period may vary from a few days or months to decades—we see a crescendo of maladjustment which is contained only by the defenses that have been described. In this unstable background, obvious and realistic factors often bring about a full-fledged attack of severe depression. These specific precipitating factors are distinct events in the life of the patient, and are not necessary in any absolute sense. However, since they occur in the most typical cases and clarify the psychodynamics of severe depression in general, I shall discuss their occurrence and import. Later we will examine the cases in which precipitating factors cannot be individuated.

The main precipitating situations may be

classified into three categories: (1) the patient's realization that his relationship with the dominant other has failed; (2) the death of the dominant other; and (3) the patient's realization of having failed in his attempt to reach a dominant goal, and his subsequent negative reevaluation of the self-image.

These situations are considered separately for didactic reasons, but they have a single and common basis: the loss of something very valuable. This "something," even if represented by a concrete situation, transcends the reality of the concrete situation. At times the loss has not yet occurred, but the knowledge that it is impending seems so certain to the patient that he experiences depression instead of anxiety. The precipitating event causes a great deal of anguish or psychological pain, which is felt very intensely for these reasons:

1. The patient's cognitive appraisal of the event leads him to realize that it will cause a disorganization of his life structure and self-image.

2. His main cognitive construct and pattern of living will no longer enable him to cope with the situation. This realization reevokes

what can be pictured as a distant but resounding echo of the pain sustained early in life, when the patient felt he had lost the love of his mother or the mother substitute. The present loss has the same value as the loss of the mother's love.

3. The patient realizes that all the methods which he used to prevent the catastrophe have failed.

4. He also believes that the methods he used were the only ones he could use or knew how to use. Thus he finds himself in a situation of helplessness. He cannot put into practice the methods used by the normal person recovering from normal sadness. For the patient, using alternative courses is an impossibility. Thus he cannot do sorrow work.

5. Instead, his sadness becomes depression, which continues to increase in intensity.

The development of these psychological events will be described in greater detail in the following sections.

Depression Following Deterioration Of The Main Interpersonal Relation

The situation in which the patient realizes the failure of his main interpersonal relation (the relation with the dominant other) is in my opinion the most typical of those which lead to severe depression. Thus it will be described in detail, the other situations, which will be examined later in this chapter, will be described only or predominantly in those aspects which differ from the situation we are now examining. Depression following deterioration of the main interpersonal relation occurs much more often in women, so I shall refer to the patient in the feminine gender. It is to be understood that the same situation takes place in a considerable number of male patients.

Events that have drastically affected the life of the patient may have occurred recently. The husband may have asked for a divorce, or may have been discovered as having an extramarital affair. Often, however, a few disparate happenings, certain decisions which have been made, or a review of one's life have induced the patient to reexamine her marital situation. At times the effect of the precipitating event was unforeseeable: reading a book, or seeing a play or a movie which revealed itself full of psychological significance for the patient. The marital partner— whom the patient considered a protector, a pillar on whom she depended entirely, a distributor of love, sex, affect, approval, food, and money—is now seen as an authoritarian person who imposes his rule at times in a subtle, hardly recognizable fashion, at other times in an obvious way. The patient's life, believed to be devoted to affection, family care, doing hard work, or the nourishment and reaffirmation of love, is now seen as a nongenuine life. The patient has denied many aspects of living because she wanted peace and approval at any cost. She has been excessively compliant, submissive, and accommodating. By always doing what the husband wanted and by denying her wishes, she has not been true to herself; as a matter of fact, she has betrayed herself. In some cases the patient may exaggerate and see the authoritarian husband as a tyrant, somebody who deserves not love but hate, somebody who wants to enslave her and change her real nature. In most cases she does not realize that she also has played a role in establishing this type of interpersonal relation. She has done so with her submissiveness and ingratiating attitude, by accepting the patriarchal model of society, or by making the dominant other believe that she was perfectly contented or even happy with this state of living. She has indeed submitted herself, bent her head, and allowed herself to be transformed against her real wishes. There is nothing wrong, of course, in adopting the husband's ways of living if the wife really wishes to do so or because she genuinely believes they are better or more adequate than her own. But if she accepts them only to placate the spouse, and if she deceives herself into thinking that she likes these changes in her way of living when she really does not, she injures herself.

The new evaluation of her husband—the kind of dominating person he really is—is not easily accepted. A normal person would accept the new appraisal, no matter how painful it was, and try to do her best with what remained of her life (separation, divorce, other affections.) But the patient cannot. She cannot bring herself to conclude that she has wasted her life. She still needs the same dominant other to praise her, approve of her, and make her feel worthwhile. How could he continue to play that role if she expressed hate, rebellion, or in some cases even self-assertion?

Thus the patient finds herself in a situation in which she cannot change her cognitive structures. She has reached a critical point at which a realignment of psychodynamic forces and a new pattern of interpersonal relationships are due, but she is not able to implement them; and this is her predicament. Often she denies her negative appraisal of the dominant other and of her life—that is, she represses her ideas—but the feeling of sadness remains conscious and is intensely experienced. Inasmuch as she cannot organize alternative structures, such as new plans for her life and new ways of evaluating herself as a person, she feels helpless. She cannot do what normal people resort to in order to solve their sorrow.

The anguish is experienced and retained, and as a rule becomes more and more pronounced. The sorrow is replaced by an overpowering wave of depression which submerges every idea. A few very painful thoughts remain. Eventually almost all ideas become unconscious and the patient is only aware of an overpowering feeling of depression. The slowing down of thought processes is also responsible for the decrease in mobility that the patient shows at this point. Movements and actions, in order to be implemented, must be preceded by ideomotor activity which is now greatly decreased. The slowing down of thought processes is, however, a self-defeating mechanism. At this point, constellations of thought continue to activate the depression even if they are unconscious. If we ask the patient why she is depressed, often she does not know.

At times a few thoughts remain as conscious, cognitive islands in the ocean of the depressive feeling. The patient may feel very guilty. The guilt is caused by emerging thoughts that offer a new evaluation of the dominant other. The patient feels guilty for seeing him in so bad a light when she used to see him as a saint to be revered and respected. In her depressed condition, she is generally not able to trace the guilt feeling; she just feels guilty and may give absurd explanations for her guilt. She has done "terrible things," and so forth. In many instances hate for the husband is not repressed to such a degree that the patient cannot feel guilty about it. On the other hand, if she were able to deal with this hate at a fully conscious level, she would be able to change the situation less inadequately. As a matter of fact, she could even realize in certain cases that her hate was too strong a feeling, and not congruous with the circumstances. But she cannot face what she believes would undermine the foundation of her life and prove the futility of all her past efforts. Thus she represses her hate and she continues to follow a pattern of silent submission. Even when she was not so sick, she did not reveal or admit to her friends the hostile feelings for her husband.

The guilt feeling to which we have referred often assumes such a predominant role as to confer to the symptomatology the picture of selfblaming depression, the manifest aspect of which was described in chapter 3. Special characteristics of the environment either facilitate or make less probable the occurrence of guilt feelings, as will be described in chapter 16. The self-blaming picture is much less frequent now than it was until the middle 1940s. Nevertheless, even at present this picture is observed quite frequently.

The guilt feelings continue in these patients a trend started in childhood, that no matter how much the patient docs to remedy the situation, it is not enough. Later she feel that it is her fault that the relationship with the dominant other has not worked out. Finally, she feels guilty, as has been described, for feeling in such a negative way toward her husband. When the patient reaches the state of severe despair and blames herself, suicidal ideas occur with progressive frequency.

The number of suicidal patients is greater in men. Thus I shall refer again to the patient in the male gender.

The patient who blames himself seems to send a message: "I do not deserve any pity, any help. I deserve to die. I should do to myself what you should do to me, but you are too good to do it."

As the suicidal ideas recur, the patient may make a suicidal attempt which in a considerable percentage of cases is successful.

At this point we must try to understand the significance of the suicidal attempt. Several hypotheses have been advanced.

1. The patient wants to punish himself.

2. He wants relief from suffering or an end to a worthless life.

3. He wants to kill symbolically the dominant other.

4. The suicide has no meaning. It is just an indication of the worsening of the biochemical alteration which brought about the depression.

In accordance with the general character of this book, we shall consider only 1, 2, and 3. The first two possibilities are self-contradictory or self-exclusive until seen from the standpoint of the emotional state of the patient. The feeling that it is better to die than to suffer so much is certainly experienced. The patient would not carry out the suicidal ideas, however, if they were not reinforced or sustained by the other idea that he deserves to die and he must inflict the supreme punishment on himself. In some cases it is possible to retrace in the patient who has attempted suicide the notion that he was making a desperate effort to redeem himself by punishing himself. Probably in a subconscious, nonverbalized way the patient feels, "Punish yourself and you will be accepted again. You are acceptable but not accepted. Forgiveness is eventually available. The intermittent love will be given again." Of course, if the patient is dead he cannot receive love, but this is a realistic consideration which he cannot conceive of at the present time. Or perhaps he believes that he will be forgiven and loved in the memory of the survivors. Thus two or more logically selfcontradictory motivations coexist and reinforce one another.

The orthodox Freudian interpretation holds that suicide represents the attempt to kill the detested person who has been incorporated—in the terminology used here, the dominant other.

As I mentioned in a previous section, the individual who is prone to this type of psychotic depression has totally accepted the Thou since his early infancy. At times he lets the Thou suffocate or smother the I. In this light, the suicidal attempt is the culmination of the process; it is the Thou who finally kills the I, not the I who kills the Thou. If the I killed the Thou, there would be a complete and sudden reversal of the previous and constant trend of self-denial. Rado (1951) ingeniously tried to solve the problem by assuming that the superego (the Thou) is divided into two parts, one which the patient wants to love and another which he wants to kill. However, I am convinced that, at least in my clinical experience, the patient really wanted to kill himself. But by killing himself he would achieve a complete acceptance or introjection of a distorted image of the Thou.

There are several other factors that support this point of view. First, many cases of suicide seem to occur not when the state of melancholia is at its peak but at an early stage of remission, when the worst is over. This characteristic may of course be interpreted in various ways. The first explanation is simple and mechanical: when the patient is very depressed, he is in or almost in a stupor; he cannot act, he is extremely slow or immobile, he cannot move or think coordinately, and therefore he cannot carry out his intentions. When he becomes less retarded and more capable of coordinating his thoughts, he goes ahead with his destructive intention. The alternative possibility is that the patient who has gone through terrible experiences at the acme of his depression is afraid that these experiences may recur and, rather than face them again, he prefers to die. (This of course corresponds to the first possibility mentioned.)

Another interpretation is possible: the patient who has a great deal of guilt feels that even the most severe depth of depression has not been enough; it has not succeeded in relieving him entirely of his guilt, and only by killing himself will he entirely redeem himself.

This last interpretation is supported by other factors. Significantly, there is almost complete relief after the suicide attempt. The Freudian interpretation would lead one to expect an increase in guilt feeling (for having attempted but not actually succeeded in killing the superego) and a consequent increase in depression. As Weiss (1957, 1974) and others have emphasized, in the attempt itself—that is, in gambling with death—the patient feels that he has been punished adequately. He has done what the Thou wanted and now he can live peacefully. Often there is no need for the suicide attempt; after having gone through the acme of his depression, the patient feels suddenly relieved, and a marked improvement occurs.

According to Kolb (1959), "The suicidal maneuver is often determined by familyindicated permission for acting out." In his clinical experience, the psychodynamic explanation of acting out which has been given for other antisocial acts is also valid for suicide: in families where suicide has occurred, the likelihood of suicide for the manic-depressive patient is much higher than otherwise. Where suicide has not occurred, one usually finds threats of suicide or intimidating actions suggesting suicide on the part of the parents.

Through many years of practice I have found, however, an increasing number of patients who did not feel guilty and yet had decided to put an end to their "worthless" lives. In several cases there was a confusion about whether the patient considered life, at least his own, or himself to be worthless. The only certainty was the horrible mental pain which had to be terminated at any cost.

The relief experienced by the patient after an acute attack of depression is remarkable. The patient feels guilt-free and accepted, and wants to settle down in his own life. Even reality seems pleasant, and he does not want to be alone; he wants to be close to the mate. This attempt, however, will not work out unless successful therapy intervenes. The patient who improves after the nadir of depression, whether or not this nadir led to a suicidal attempt, eventually will feel depressed again. The relatively free interval may last a few hours, days, weeks, months, or longer.

The improvement or depression-free interval is susceptible to several hypothetical interpretations. One is that the patient feels he has expiated his guilt. However, another one seems to me more plausible and consonant with what several patients in psychotherapy have told me. An idea presents itself which somehow succeeds in cutting the main line of depressogenic cognition and flashing a lesser, more hopeful, but secondary cognitive structure. This lesser structure may have always existed or, more seldom, have been provided by an unexpected external event. The secondary cognitive structure in some cases may be organized and increased to the point of offering considerable relief. In many cases, however, the predominant depressogenic structure tends to acquire the upper hand and the patient becomes depressed again.

In some untreated cases the depression may become chronic and severe; in others it remains chronic but less severe; and finally, it may alternate between being severe and mild. At the present stage of knowledge we cannot be absolutely sure why some untreated cases of severe depression become intermittent, improve, or even recover. For some unpredictable reasons they eventually become capable of escaping from the rigid cognitive construct and finding alternative patterns.

Some patients, especially those who could be classified as suffering from manic-depressive psychosis, are able to change the depression into a manic, hypomanic, or mini-manic attack.

In the manic attack the Thou is not eliminated or projected to the external world; it is only disregarded. The patient must continue to force himself into a distracted and frenzied mood which shuts out not only introspection, but any well-organized thinking. In the manic state there is no elimination of the Freudian superego, as perhaps there is in some psychopaths. The superego is very much present, and the manic frenzy is a method of dealing with it.

But neither the depression nor the manic attack actually bring about a solution to the deeply rooted conflicts. Even after having paid the penalty of the severe attack, many patients (but not all) will have a more or less free interval and then tend to be affected again by the same difficulty, which will be channeled into the same pattern—with the cycle likely to repeat itself. Moreover we must realize that this type of depression, as well as all the others that shall be discussed in this book, becomes the fundamental and habitual mode of living. As we shall discuss later, the patient selects depressive thoughts (Beck's depressive triad) to sustain the familiar mood. Little disappointments, losses, or accidental happenings that lead the patient to self-accusation, guilt, or severe depression are actually symbolic of an earlier and greater disappointment, or of lifelong disappointment. Kraepelin (1921), to show the relative unimportance of psychogenic factors, reported a woman who had three attacks of depression: the first after the death of her husband, the second after the death of her dog, and the third after the death of her dove. From what has been discussed so far, it is apparent that each of these deaths was not necessarily traumatic per se. One may guess that the death of the dove reactivated the sorrow the patient had experienced at the previous deaths, and it was also symbolic of a much greater loss, perhaps of the meaning or purpose in her life.

So far I have interpreted psychodynamically

attacks of severe depression caused by the realization of the failure of an important interpersonal relation, as in the case of a patient who follows a pattern of submission and placation in her relation with a dominant other. The patient who instead follows a pattern of dependency and eventually develops a symptomatology of the claiming type, at a certain point in her life realizes that she no longer can depend on this interpersonal relationship. Without being aware of it, to a considerable extent she still is claiming the lost paradise or the bliss of the early life when she was completely dependent on the duty-bound mother or mother substitute. As the patient makes herself dependent on the dominant other and becomes more demanding, she feels more deprived. Any unfulfilled demand is experienced as a wound, a serious deprivation, an insult, or an irreparable loss, and it brings about an unpleasant feeling of sadness which cannot be solved and is followed by depression.

The new way of experiencing the relationship with the dominant other is based on the fact that the affect or love which reassured her and in whose name she expected a great deal is now recognized as uncertain, insincere, unreliable, about to finish, or finished already. She too does not love the husband anymore, and therefore she feels she cannot expect much from him. The sad reality, however, is that she depends on him psychologically, economically, and socially, and she cannot do without him. Like the previous type of patient that I described, she finds herself in a trap from which she cannot escape. She becomes more and more depressed and suicidal. In these cases the suicide attempt seems to convey the message, "Do not abandon me. You have the power to prevent my death. You will feel guilty if you don't give me what I need and let me die." However, there is a feeling of hopelessness, the feeling that the dominant other will not listen to this appeal and will let her down. For a certain number of patients in this category the dominant other is not the spouse, but one or both parents. Many patients have always remained dependent on their parents. Although they would like to be free of them to go on their own, be self-supporting, and get married, they cannot. They are caught again in a vicious cycle from which they cannot escape (dependency and resentment or hate for the persons on whom they depend). Perhaps more than any other patients, they represent those described by Abraham who, as a consequence of early love deprivation, remain fixated at oral erotism and maintain a general dependency on people.

Depression Following Death, Loss, Or Disappearance Of The Dominant Other

In these cases depression occurs when the dominant other is no longer available. The most common cause is death. Cases involving divorce will not be considered here because the separation was caused by a failure of the interpersonal relation, and these cases are therefore included in the previously described category. However, some cases in which one spouse suddenly abandons the other, gives ultimatums, or unexpectedly declares his intention to dissolve the marriage may represent a mixture of the two categories.

Less common precipitating factors of severe depression are loss of friendship, companionship, affection, or approval because a person close to the patient moved away or got married and had to exclude the patient or relegate him to a minor role.

Contrary to the typical cases in the first

category, the patient at a conscious level does not feel abandoned by the dominant other on account of failure in the relationship; rather, it is because of circumstances beyond his control such as death or moving to a distant location for reasons of work. Whether the patient considers these causes legitimate is debatable: in most cases there is no doubt that at least unconsciously the patient considers the dominant other responsible for leaving, even if he left because he died. He should not have allowed himself to die. There is also no doubt that some patients feel, even at a conscious level, responsible for the disappearance or death of the dominant other. If they had treated him better, he would not have died. Instead the bad behavior of the patient has made the dominant other unhappy and sick or more likely to die. Thus the patient has "killed" him or her.

In other cases the patient feels guilty because in moments of reemerging resentment he recognizes that he wished the death of the lost person. The wish has now become reality: to the wish is attributed the primitive power of engendering reality. The patient accuses himself of having entertained the murderous desire.

All these interpretations connected with guilt are derivatives of Freud's concept that guilt and self-depreciation are diverted anger which was directed originally toward the love object (our dominant other). As I have already mentioned, however, guilt does not seem to play such an important role as it did once. Perhaps it will reacquire importance in the future.

Bemporad (1970) has advanced another explanation. The patient, who was totally dependent on the dominant other for selfesteem, acceptance, approval, and appreciation, realizes that he cannot depend on him any more. And yet he is incapable of "autonomous gratification," of supplying what he needs to himself. He becomes sad and then depressed because of being deprived of this gratification. In other words, the depression is the result of

deprivation (emotional and cognitive).

Bemporad's interpretation is valid in some cases of severe depression, as well, but with support from other factors that complicate the picture. First, I must stress that for the reasons illustrated earlier in this chapter, the patient is

incapable of finding cognitive-affective

alternatives to what was provided by the former dominant other. Second, the patient does not want to believe that the dominant other could be substituted. He rejects the possibility because to admit it would be tantamount to conceding that the dominant other was not indispensable in the first place. This conclusion, if accepted, would require a reassessment of the patient's whole life and might induce a state of panic that the patient cannot even contemplate. Thus he is still motivated to think that the dominant other was indispensable and irreplaceable. Whenever reality indicates the opposite—that life can be worthwhile even without the dominant other — such possibility is assessed in a distorted way, appears threatening, and may bring about further depression.

Depression Following Realization Of Failing To Reach The Dominant Goal

This type of depression occurs among men more frequently than depressions which follow other patterns, but in terms of absolute incidence this depression too is more frequent among women. The goal most frequently experienced by women as not achieved or notto-be-achieved is romantic love. Being unloved for them means being unlovable. Thus what is disturbing is not only the lack of the joy of love, but the injury to the self-image. However, the cultural and social changes which are rapidly taking place in the status of women have already diminished the frequency of unachieved love as the precipitating factor of severe depression. To be exact, love does remain an important precipitating factor when it is lost, as described in the previous category. It is less frequently the precipitating factor of severe depression in the role of a dominant goal which has not been achieved.

In men the dominant goal which most frequently precipitates a severe depression, because it is experienced as not achieved or not to be achieved, has to do with work and career. Here too, the most traumatic part of this realization is in what it does to the self-image. Certainly the patient is very interested in his career and work, but the depressive elements are his cognitive ramifications—mostly unconscious or only dimly conscious—that associate work and career with what he and others think of him, and with his being a worthwhile person and deserving love. Now he has come to the realization that he is not going to be a great lawyer, doctor, politician, actor, writer, lover, industrialist, inventor, musician, and so forth. He cannot go into another field or give up his ambition because his whole life has been centered on the achievement of this particular goal. Nothing else counts: after this dramatic realization, life seems worthless to him; as a matter of fact, it seems painful and hard to endure.

If he wanted to be a great conductor—a Toscanini—now he has to face the fact that he is not a Toscanini; he is himself, John Doe. But he has no respect for John Doe, and he believes John Doe is nothing. There is some justification in the patient's assessment of himself in this negative way because he spent so much of his thoughts and daydreams in being a Toscanini, and his psychological life without this overpowering fantasy seems empty. Thus we must realize that the depression is not only a mourning of a fantasy; it is the mourning of a large part of one's life spent at the service of a fantasy. This explains why the depression can reach such depth and be so persistent.

This sequence of thought processes and accompanying negative feelings is made possible by the limitations of the patient, by his inability to find solutions. At times the patient may visualize alternatives, but they seem to him either unsurmountable or not worthwhile. The inability to shift to different ways of living is not due to congenital defect or to lack of intelligence, but is only the result of a life history characterized by rigid adherence to those life patterns that were described earlier in this chapter. This inability of which the patient is often unconscious can be overcome totally or to a large extent by proper psychotherapy.

In some cases the psychodynamic picture is more complicated. The patient feels that he has not been true to himself, or he has not run after the goal in the right way. For instance, he wanted to be a great conductor like Toscanini, but instead he pursued business, money, women, and so on. Now he finds himself trapped: his sadness has become a severe depression from which he does not know how to rescue himself.

Special Cases And Conclusions

Cases that do not fit exactly into the previously mentioned categories but which partake of some of their characteristics are very frequent. I shall mention the most common combinations. The depression may occur after the patient has been dismissed from an institution, organization, or company to which he devoted the prime of his life. This disappointment is often experienced as due to the loss of employment. As a matter of fact, Malzberg (1940) found that during the economic depression of 1929 to 1937 the effect of loss of employment or financial loss was statistically evident in manic-depressive patients. In 1933, for instance, 26.2 percent of first admission patients in New York state hospitals who were diagnosed as manic-depressive presented loss of employment or financial loss as the precipitating factor, whereas in the same year only 9.6 percent of first admission patients with the diagnosis of dementia praecox (schizophrenia) presented financial loss as a precipitating factor.

In some cases, not dismissal but failure to obtain a promotion is the precipitating factor. In these cases the trauma is sustained partially as a loss of a nonpersonal dominant other, and partially as failure to reach or retain the dominant goal. The source of gratification is lost as well as a gratifying self-image that the patient could maintain only through his association with that particular organization.

Depression, often leading to suicide, occurs quite frequently in unmarried men after retirement. They feel suddenly deprived of their only aspect of gratification. In women, depressions occur frequently, but not as frequently as they used to, during or about the time of the menopause, as we shall see in greater detail in chapter 12.

Depressions occur relatively frequently in twins, especially female identical twins. Although my statistics are very limited, I can say that I have found nothing specific in these cases except the psychological picture derived from being a twin. Generally one of the twins assumes the role of the dominant other and the other takes on the submissive or dependent role. The dominant other plays the role of leader, teacher, and mentor; the submissive twin plays the role of the follower, pupil, and child. In these cases the parents have played a secondary role because of their advanced age, detachment, illness, or geographical distance; and they have always remained pale figures, thus permitting one twin to acquire a parental or dominant role. When the dominant twin withdraws his support, or gets married, or separates from the submissive twin, the latter undergoes a severe trauma, experiences a feeling of helplessness, and often becomes depressed.

Less typical but more frequent, especially among females, are cases in which two siblings, not twins but close in age, live in the same dyad of dominant-dominated. In these cases the parents also have played a parental role which has been less effective than usual and which has been assumed in quite an inappropriate manner by the dominant sibling. The submissive sibling tends to become depressed whenever there is a disruption in his relation with the dominant sibling or whenever he has to revise the image of the sibling which he has incorporated.

In some patients an attack apparently is precipitated not by a loss, but by what may even seem a pleasant event. For instance, women in their forties or fifties who may have undergone previous subliminal attacks of depression can develop a severe attack shortly after the marriage of an only son or daughter. Here the event is experienced by the patient not as something pleasant but as a loss. The child whom the mother needed so much, and who was her only purpose and satisfaction in life, is now abandoning her.

In other cases an attack occurs after a promotion, which is interpreted by the patient as a new imposition that he is unable to cope with. The patient is tired of new duties and, furthermore, the new position with its added responsibility removes the security the patient had established with painstaking effort. In other cases the individual who is faced with promotion dreads the expected envy and rage of previous associates to whom he is closely bound. The expectation of such emotions in others separates him from them and thus leads to feelings of loneliness and depression. In all these cases there is difficulty in abandoning the old patterns of living which conferred security to the patient, and inability to find alternatives suitable to the new conditions.

If we now try to abstract from all the human conditions that we have described in this chapter what leads to a severe depression, we can say that it is the experience of a loss of what seems to the patient the most valuable or meaningful aspect of his life. Even more crucial is the feeling of being unable to retrieve or substitute what has been lost.

At times the severe sorrow of the depressed

person acts also as a representation of what was lost, because as long as the sorrow remains, the loss is not complete. In these cases the sorrow is like the faint image of a lost hope, the shadow of the absent, the echo of a voice heard repeatedly —perhaps with ambiguous resonance, but also with some affection, respect, and love.

At other times, implicit in the experience of loss, is the feeling that life has become unworthy or meaningless. At still other times the patient realizes that the meaning he has given to his life is inappropriate or unworthy, but if he renounces that meaning his life sustains the greatest possible loss: it becomes meaningless. His pain bespeaks his refusal to see life in that way.

Notes

[12] Some statistical works, however, seem to indicate that the first born child is more liable to manic-depressive psychosis. Of course the first-born child also is more liable to be displaced. Berman (1933) in a study of 100 manic depressives found that 48 were first-born, 15 second, 10 each third and fourth, and 17 fifth or later. Pollock and coworkers (1939) found that 39.7 percent were first-born and 29.7 percent were second-born. Malzberg (1937) and Katz (1934) could not find any relationship between birth order and manic-depressive psychosis.

[13] As is customary in English, I refer to the general patient as *he* and consider him in his male role. However, as I shall mention

later in this chapter, women with this type of personality are more numerous than men. In some special situations which are described later, in which women outnumber men by far—at least in the ratio of two to one—I shall refer to the patient by using the feminine gender.

[7]

PSYCHODYNAMICS OF MILD DEPRESSION

Jules Bemporad

In contrast to the individuals described in the previous chapter, those to be considered in this chapter are not so impaired that the affect of depression overwhelms all other psychic contents. They actively want to be rid of their feelings of depression and try to fight them off. These patients attempt to reestablish the pathological equilibrium that they had achieved prior to being depressed. They do not collapse in the face of overwhelming despair so that their psychic life is devoid of all content except for the repetitive painful ruminations which enhance the misery of their affliction. These individuals, while depressed, manage to function in their everyday lives, albeit often in a reduced capacity. They are capable of reasoning and normal cognitive abilities, and an insight-oriented approach to therapy may rapidly be initiated. Some somatic symptoms such as anorexia or insomnia may be present but are not pronounced. Psychomotor retardation and constipation are not seen, but loss of libido is not uncommon. Most significant, perhaps, is that these less severely depressed individuals maintain their relationships to others: in fact, they may frantically search for comfort and support from other people. They do not withdraw from interpersonal relationships into a silent world of solitary suffering.

Such individuals are typified by the presence of the affect of depression which may be constant or fluctuate in intensity. As will be further discussed, this sense of mental anguish may take a variety of forms— from an agonizing awareness of loss to a despairing conclusion that life is pointless and lacks any form, purpose, or meaning. Regardless of the cognitive variations, the basic mood of depression is definitely present. Before proceeding with an analysis of such individuals, it may be worthwhile to consider the conceptual status of depression as an affect as I view it, since this view naturally will influence the interpretation of depressed patients.

As described in chapter 2, the psychodynamic interpretation of depression has undergone numerous transformations in the history of psychoanalytic thought. Some authors have attempted to explain the experience of depression as a complex metapsychological phenomenon, such as an aggressive cathexis of the self-representation, or as a conflict between the punishing superego and the helpless ego.

Others have presented the less complicated position that depression is actually a primary affect that cannot further be reduced to more basic constructs. I definitely lean toward this latter conceptualization and agree with Sandler and Joffe's (1965) statement that "if depression is viewed as an affect, if we allot to it the same conceptual status as the affect of anxiety, then much of the literature on depression in childhood (and this could be extended to adults) can be integrated in a meaningful way" (p. 90).

[14]

However, considering depression as a primary affect does not automatically imply that it is a simple emotion devoid of complex cognitive components. As indicated by Arieti in chapter 5, different emotions presuppose a greater or lesser cognitive maturity and intellectual understanding. Depression appears to be a third-order emotion necessitating some awareness of the past and the future, some linguistic ability, and some recognition of the effects of human beings on one another. This particular painful feeling automatically arises whenever the individual "senses" that he has either irrevocably lost or never will achieve a needed state of well-being of the self. I have put the word senses in quotes because this awareness is not necessarily explicit; rather, it is the unconscious cognitive system that seems to give rise to emotion. By unconscious cognitive system I mean a structure of aspirations, fears, and general expectations from the self and from others that guide the individual's behavior but of which he may not be explicitly aware. These systems of belief are postulated to be at a different level of consciousness than the superficial pessimistic distortions which occur subsequent to the onset of a depressive episode. These deeper cognitive systems are the cause rather than the result of the manifest experience of depression and are not so readily available to being clearly spelled out in conscious awareness.

For example, an individual may become depressed after a loss but remain unclear as to the manner in which the loss has affected him.

Similarly, other individuals may become depressed without any precipitating environmental trauma or without knowing why they should experience a sense of dysphoria at this particular time of their lives. Freud (1917) astutely noted this lack of awareness: he observed that even when the melancholic relates his plight as resulting from the loss of someone, "he knows whom he has lost but not *what* it is he has lost in them." What has been lost is an environmental prop that allowed the perpetuation of a needed state of self. The depressive does not appear to grieve for the other; rather, he grieves for himself—for being deprived of what the other had supplied. He grieves over his state of self without the other or without his all-important goal (as seen in socalled reactive depressions). Or the individual may grieve over a state of self that finds no meaning or gratification in life, unaware that his unconscious cognitive system has forced him to inhibit himself so that he shuns meaningful achievement or pleasurable activities (as seen in so-called characterological depressions).

The philosopher Kierkegaard was well aware that the true cause of despair is despair about one's own self, regardless of the apparently precipitating events. He wrote that "when the ambitious man whose watchword as 'either Caesar or nothing' does not become Caesar, he is in despair thereat. But this signifies something else, namely, that precisely because he did not become Caesar he cannot endure to be himself" (1954, p. 152). In describing depression resulting from an environmental loss, Kierkegaard observed:

> A young girl is in despair over love and so she despairs over her lover, because he died, or because he was unfaithful to her .... No, she is in despair over herself. This self of hers, if it had become "his" beloved, she would have been rid of in the most blissful way, or would have lost, this self is now a torment to her when it has to be a self without "him" (1954, p. 153)

Kierkegaard beautifully and concisely revealed the self-centered aspect of depression as well as its cause that ultimately resides in the deprivation of something which is needed to transform the self and to give the self a sense of worth and well-being, whether this something is the achievement of an ambition, a continued relationship with a needed other, or the maintenance of a particular mode of life.

Therefore depression may be conceptualized as a complex emotion that arises when an individual is deprived (or deprives himself) of an element of life that is necessary for a satisfactory state of self. However, most if not all mature individuals experience such episodes of mental pain during their lives without becoming clinically depressed. Some marshall their inner resources and continue to press on for fulfillment with renewed hope. Others tolerate the shattering of their wished-for state of self and readjust their aspirations or seek other avenues of meaning. Still others do not give in to their depression but defend against it by various external or internal means: external defenses are usually drugs or alcohol, and internal means are commonly states of depersonalization or an obsession with hypochondriacal concerns. Many individuals, however, progress from the initial depressive psychobiological reaction as described by Sandler and Joffe (1965) to a true clinical depression. These individuals are predisposed to depressive attacks; that is, they have a particular premorbid personality which leaves them vulnerable to repeated bouts of depression. These pathological personality patterns are always present; so that depression has been described by some authors, such a Bonime (1962), as a practice, a way of life, rather than a periodic illness with healthy intervals. According to this view, Bonime has further implied that the predisposed individual decompensates when his maladaptive interpersonal transactions are no longer effective in bolstering a specious sense of self. This position can be widened to include the role of one's concept of self and others in the role of depression. When such a concept either obviates the possibility of meaning or is transformed by a loss or frustration so that meaning is no longer possible, depression ensues.

Types of Mild Depression

As previously indicated, mild (or dystonic) forms of depression may be classified into three major types: reactive, characterological, and masked. The symptoms of these varieties have been described in chapter 3. Here the discussion will focus on the underlying psychodynamics of these varieties first. The reactive and characterological depressions will be considered. The major clinical differentiation between these two types is that the former occurs after an identifiable and subjectively severe trauma in the individual's life and the latter is exhibited in a chronically ungratifying form of existence.

The reactive forms of depression have already been described in detail and their exposition will not be repeated here. The differences between individuals who develop a severe depression following the loss of a dominant other or frustration in the attainment of a dominant goal, and those who respond to such subjective traumas with only mild or moderate feelings of depression, may lie in the quality and relative quantity of pathological beliefs.

Most, but by no means all severe depressives appear to have utilized the dominant other or dominant goal in order somehow to absolve themselves from a sense of inner evil or badness. In contrast, the individual who suffers from a milder form of depression does not uniformly see himself as evil, but utilizes the dominant other or goal to obtain pleasure and meaning. The search is not to eradicate a negative; rather, it is to add a positive aspect to life. Obviously each situation is more complicated, consisting of a mixture of relative absolution and satisfaction to be derived from others. However, in my experience, individuals suffering from milder forms of depression do not give protestations of personal malevolence or baseness. They may see themselves as deprived, lazy, helpless, or at fault for their loss, but the malignant undercurrent of true self-vilification (not a specious self-blame in order to manipulate others) is usually absent.

Another difference is the degree to which the dominant other or goal has completely monopolized the person's life. Severe depressives appear to derive their total sense of self from some external agency. Less afflicted individuals, while showing an inordinate need for the other or for the goal to serve vital psychic functions, are able to develop other—-albeit embryonic—forms of obtaining self-esteem. In terms of cognitive beliefs, mildly depressed individuals appear to be better able to discover alternatives in their modes of thought. They are less rigidly bound to one set of ideas which govern all validations of the self. For example, these individuals are able to shift their attention rapidly to the therapist in the hope of reestablishing a pathological relationship. In contrast to severe depressives, they are not bound to so limited a cast of characters from whom to derive meaning. (Other differences between these two groups are presented at the end of this chapter.)

The term chronic depression is meant to describe two general types of patients. One group has a similar psychic structure to the reactive group but differs in that the relationship with a dominant other or the pursuit of a goal does not consistently or adequately dissipate feelings of depression. The other group is chronically depressed as a result of unrealistic standards that result from irrational beliefs of the self and others and which prevent satisfaction or pleasure in life. Both groups share a consistent lack of joyfulness in life, a low estimate of self, and an oversensitivity to minor environmental frustrations or to trivial negative reactions of others. Most significantly, both groups endure periods of depression of varying intensity. This painful affect is a constant undertone to daily existence, during which it is at times more or less pronounced. This sense of depression, joylessness, and at times even of despair is multidetermined but most immediately results from a stifling self-inhibition of pleasurable activities and a fear of other people's reactions which the depressive often distorts or magnifies.

The first group appears to inhibit normal pleasurable activities for fear of losing the dominant other or because such activities may interfere with the attainment of a dominant goal. In this former case, the cause of inhibition may appear to be initiated externally. However, there is actually an internal restriction of activities since the individual will project all sorts of prohibitions on others in the environment. His fantasied restrictions are often more severe than the dominant other would impose. Similarly, in the latter case the individual erroneously believes that, as if by some sort of malevolent magic, any momentary diversion or pleasure will threaten his quest for the all-embracing goal. Such individuals are in a precarious situation since any sign of disapproval (real or imagined) from a glorified other or any subjectively believed impasse to obtaining a significant goal will result in prolonged periods of depression.

The second, or inhibited, group does not appear to experience depression directly as a result of environmental events. Rather, these individuals suffer from a chronic sense of futility and hopelessness because they do not allow themselves to become actively involved in rewarding activities. They often superficially exhibit a sense of prideful and moralistic superiority that covers a quite infantile personality which is scrupulously hidden from others. Evidences of this underlying pathology are the almost paranoid belief that others watch their every move, and their secret wishes to be passively taken care of by powerful others. These individuals dread the exposure of their dependency needs or the public expression of free, spontaneous behavior. They live ascetic, unfulfilled lives, imagine that others are keeping track of their behavior (as their parents had done), and suppress healthy desires for closeness and mutuality. The mode of existence that such structures impose becomes chronically dissatifying and eventually devoid of meaning. These individuals may gradually become so removed from true involvement in life that their unsatisfied needs become forgotten and they simply feel an inner emptiness or feel cut off from the world. In some depressives this inner emptiness may be temporarily abated by alcohol or drugs which can offer only short-term relief.

From afar, these individuals appear to be paragons of success and proper adjustment as well as of psychological maturity. It is in the course of therapy that they begin to recognize and reveal not only the extent of their depression, but also the well of unsatisfied yearnings that they have shunned since childhood. They also demonstrate the presence of rigid, inflexible beliefs about themselves and others which prevent fulfillment in life. This strict code of conduct exacts its price in terms of closeness, pleasure, and meaning. In later life they may see through the irrationality of their behavior but be unable to bring themselves to change without the aid of therapy. They see themselves caught in a way of life that no longer brings even the bogus self-satisfaction of alleged moral superiority. Yet there is no awareness of how they can alter their beliefs by themselves. The old parental "shoulds" have lost their former rationality but not their tyrannical power.

Masked depression presents somewhat of an enigma since the concept implies a diagnosis of depression without the major symptom of this disorder—a conscious feeling of depression. However, as described in chapter 3, various authors have maintained that patients who are addicts, have psychosomatic disorders, are accident-prone, or have other behavioral abnormalities are actually hiding an underlying depression. Lesse (1974, 1977), who has contributed extensively on this condition, wrote that "usually the depressive core surfaces spontaneously with the passage of time in a manner comparable to an iceberg that may rise to the surface under certain climactic conditions" (1977, p. 186). He believes that masked depression is a common condition that is often missed by the untrained clinician. He found that over 30 percent of depressives whom he saw as consultant to a medical unit had masked depression. Others, including myself, have found this condition to be rather rare. The frequency with which masked depressions are encountered may depend on the sample of patients seen, whether in a private psychiatric office or on the wards of medical services.

Part of the disparity in the reported frequency of masked depression also may reflect the definition of depression as well as diagnostic criteria. For example, I believe a depressed person who drinks or takes drugs should not be considered to be a masked depressive. Such a patient's depression is quite conscious and is being reduced by external factors. In contrast, an individual with an incapacitating medical illness or a serious psychiatric problem who experiences an understandable state of depression secondarily, as a reaction to his predicament, would not be classified as primarily depressed. In fact, most patients who request therapy for a variety of complaints are unhappy because their defenses or character adaptations are no longer effective. However, these individuals also would not be called depressed. In therapy such individuals describe different psychodynamics, life histories, modes of interaction, and cognitive distortions. An additional note of caution may be warranted: a large number of patients may become transiently depressed in the course of therapy as they become aware of some disagreeable aspect of themselves or have to relinquish gratifying yet neurotic behavior patterns. For example, an hysterical patient may suffer a temporary feeling of depression when he stops utilizing denial to a massive extent and takes a realistic look at his life. This does not mean that a hidden, masked depression was present all along; rather, the affect corresponds to a new and possibly healthier way of seeing reality. The process of working through may sometimes be quite painful.

With these provisos in mind, it cannot be doubted that cases of masked depression do exist. In my experience these are truly depressed patients who utilize certain defenses against the unpleasant affect just as other patients evolve methods of eliminating the experience of anxiety. These patients usually present hypochondriacal complaints which absorb their every waking moment. They are so involved with their physical state of health that they apparently manage to fight off feelings of depression. Yet even in these patients some of the familiar depressive symptomatology is present: they are sure they will never get well, they are fearful of novelty and enjoyment, they utilize symptoms to greatly inhibit their behavior, and they manipulate others by their alleged ill health.

Another type of true masked depression I have seen is the rare instance of depersonalization. In these patients the affect of depression is so painful that they cut off all feelings as a way of avoiding experiencing it. As noted in chapter 3, these patients often experience rather severe and incapacitating depression when they do not depersonalize, and it may be questioned whether they should be considered mild depressives. On the other hand, they do try to fight off the affect of depression and do not realign their cognitions so that the depression is seen as justified. They pay a great price for this defensive warding off of depression but the toll becomes understandable when they reveal the depth of their despair in the safety of the therapeutic situation. I have treated one such patient over a period of about five years. She initially had episodes of feeling empty, during which her body did not seem normal and she sensed herself as apart from the rest of the world. This woman had recurrent dreams of a terribly misshapen child whom no one could ever help. The affect in these dreams was extreme despair. In addition, she gave a history that was typical of depressed patients. As she became stronger in therapy, she was able to see the dream image as a distorted childhood estimation of herself and to confront the depressive affect related to this cognitive construct.

The status of masked depression is still unsettled since clear-cut diagnostic criteria have not been delineated and different authors may use this diagnosis liberally or very conservatively. While I lean toward the latter direction, such individuals do exist and successful treatment depends on recognizing the depressive core of their illness.

All types of mild depression share certain

psychodynamic and cognitive features beyond the manifest experience of a dysphoric affect which links them together as variations of a basic disorder. These underlying characteristics will be elaborated in the following sections in order to define the basis for the spectrum of clinical phenotypes of depression. Each factor may be relatively more or less prominent in different individuals, but the totality of these characteristics form a multifactorial network of beliefs and attitudes that predispose an individual to depressive episodes.

Restriction Of Sources Of Self-Esteem

Pathologic dependency is perhaps the one characteristic of the depressive that has been unanimously emphasized in the psychiatric literature. It was most probably this tenacious, demanding quality of melancholics that suggested to Abraham, in his pioneering work on depression, the existence of a libidinal regression to the oral stage. Although many authors have subsequently disregarded Abraham's formulations of unconscious dynamics, there has been a uniform acceptance of his excellent descriptions of the depressive's mode of object relations and character structure. Later authors have echoed the theme of dependency as central in depression, although they consider this characteristic from vastly different theoretical positions. Arieti (1962) has especially stressed the role of dependency in the etiology of depression. He noted that in his experience, decompensation of the depressive often occurs following the failure to maintain an ongoing relationship with a significant environmental figure. In contrast to the schizophrenic, in whom the psychotic transformation is in reaction to a failure of "cosmic magnitude involving the relation with the whole interpersonal world" (p. 401), depression seems to result from the loss of a relationship with one highly esteemed person in the immediate environment. Arieti calls this idealized figure the "dominant other." who regardless of substitution in adult life is symbolic of the depriving mother.

Jacobson (1971) described a similar interpersonal situation, although she utilized a different terminology in recounting her treatment of a young woman who had been subject to recurrent depressions. In formulating the dynamics of this case, Jacobson observed:

> Hence her love objects represented glorified parental images with which she identified

> through participation in their superiority. To be loved and to find recognition by them served the purpose of supporting her selfesteem, which was forever threatened by the overstrictness of her standards and the intensity of her ambitions. It is significant that Peggy (i.e. the patient) did not "borrow" the ego or superego of her love objects, as certain schizophrenics will do. What she needed was respect for them, and love, praise, and emotional support from them (1971, p. 224).

This last point is extremely important in that the depressive does not "merge" with the dominant other; he retains his own identity. However, the depressive will misuse the dominant other in order to maintain self-esteem. The dominant other structures the life of the depressive in the areas of gratification and selfworth but not so globally as in the symbiosis seen in schizophrenia.

Becker (1964) called attention to limited areas of esteem as being a significant determinant of depression. In comparing depression with schizophrenia, Becker wrote, "The depressed person, on the other hand, suffers instead from a too uncritical participation in a limited range of monopolizing interpersonal experiences" (1964, p. 131).

Becker cited Volkart's (1957) study of

bereavement which showed that pathological mourning seems to occur when the bereft has limited his sources of gratification to too few objects:

> Any culture which, in the name of mental health, encourages extreme and exclusive emotional investments by one person in a selected few others, but does not provide suitable outlets and alternatives for the inevitable bereavement, is simply altering the conditions of, and perhaps postponing, severe mental illness. It may, in the vernacular, be building persons up for a big letdown by exacerbating vulnerability (Volkart, 1957, p. 304).

Certain individuals by virtue of their upbringing appear to develop too narrow a range of activities that can supply self-esteem and thus they are vulnerable to depression if their limited number of objectives are not realized. As mentioned in chapter 6, for some the objective is the achievement of a dominant goal; for others the objective is to receive love and praise from a dominant other.

It may be noted that, contrary to the early classical formulation of depression, the predisposed individual does not create an ego introject of the mother following a loss in infancy. The internalization of parental values does not mean the incorporation of a lost love object as initially intended by Freud. Certainly all children adopt certain values and attitudes of their parents in the course of normal development without becoming depressives in adult life. The difficulty with the different meanings of internalization may be the result of a lack of reconciliation between the Freudian theory of depression and the later conceptualization of the superego. In the former, the infant incorporates the parent; in the latter, the child identifies with the parent as a solution to the Oedipal conflict. However, it is possible that internalization of parental values occurs as a gradual process throughout childhood and the concept of an introject is an unnecessary reification. More recent psychoanalytic contributions that stress infantile superego precursors seem to postulate just this preoedipal acceptance of parental attitudes without having to hypothesize the formation of a pathological introject.

Further clarification of the process of internalization also may be needed. The difference between imitative learning, whereby the child models himself after the parent, and reactive learning, whereby the child is coerced to become an idealized model desired by the parent, should be specified in reference to such terms as self-image and superego. In the case of imitative learning, the self is automatically modeled after an esteemed environmental figure, often without any underlying conflict. Reactive learning as intended here is the process whereby the child is made to become a desired ideal which does not necessarily resemble the parent, in order to win love or escape punishment. The attainment of this parental ideal leads to a sense of satisfaction not because of any inherent gratifying quality, but because it ensures parental favor.

The depressive appears to be the product of excessive reactive learning and to have developed a reactive identity; that is, he functions best in a role that reflects the dictates of dominant other rather than any independent standards. These individuals require the presence of an external agency in order to derive satisfaction, and they are unable to gain pleasure from independent achievement.

Fear Of Autonomous Gratification

Patients often exhibit a marked inability and even dread of obtaining self-esteem or pleasure through their own efforts rather than by means of a dominant other. I have found this type of pathological functioning, which may be called the fear of autonomous gratification, to be a consistent feature of depressives. This characteristic may not always be immediately apparent, especially in view of the impressive achievements of some depressives. However, on further investigation it is found that social or professional accomplishment bring the depressive little pleasure in themselves: they are sought in an attempt to win love and acceptance from an external agency or to affirm an irrational sense of self that still follows parental dictates.

Nancy, a highly successful executive who began psychotherapy after years of visiting internists with vague pains and insomnia, exemplified this fear of autonomous gratification. Although she held a position of considerable importance and made an attractive salary, she could not bring herself to furnish her apartment comfortably or live in a manner commensurate with her income. She considered anything spent on herself to be a shameful extravagance, but would buy inordinately expensive gifts for her parents. Nancy was equally self-sacrificing with her free time and canceled social engagements if her boss asked her to work late or if her father asked to see her. In actuality Nancy was unable to enjoy a social evening unless she could somehow relate it to her work, just as she had to justify buying clothes by saying that she had to dress well for work. She found it difficult to date and dreaded sexual confrontation. When she did go out, she tried to structure the evening so that she would be part of a group and thus escape being alone with a man. Even then she had to drink a good deal in order to fight feelings of guilt and degradation. Eventually Nancy confessed that even her work, which seemed to be her major concern in life, brought her no pleasure in itself but only served as a means of pleasing her boss. Whenever she gained recognition from him or when she was praised by her father, Nancy became ecstatic with a great sense of well-being and felt vibrant and alive.

Although she had been subject to mild depressive episodes for most of her life, Nancy became clinically depressed when her boss decided to retire. She felt betrayed by his leaving after her many years of self-sacrifice. This sense of desertion was intensified by her parents' coincidental plan to take an extended vacation overseas. Nancy felt that her only means of gratification and meaning were abandoning her, and the prospect of life without them was unbearable. Never having been able to gain a sense of self-esteem from her own efforts, but only through the presence of a dominant other, her life now seemed empty and pointless.

Nancy's early history can be briefly outlined. Her mother was described as a shy, helpless woman living in fear of her husband, who tyrannically ruled the household. Nancy was not allowed to form extrafamilial attachments, but was coerced to work hard and study arduously in order to bring honor to the family. She was sent to strict parochial schools and her work was closely supervised by her father, who made her feel guilty and ashamed if she did not perform according to his aspirations. She was repeatedly told how her parents were sacrificing themselves for her and how she frivolously squandered their hard-earned savings by not studying enough or by wanting to enjoy herself with school friends. Nancy grew up determined to win her father's admiration and to redeem herself against his accusations. She reacted to any activities that were not directed toward this goal with apprehension and anxiety, although she superficially disparaged them as childish and immoral. In keeping with this "pleasure anxiety," Spiegel (1959) commented that the depressive fears the experience of happiness and pleasure as much as the experience of anger. The only thing that matters is to be passively gratified by the dominant other, to be reassured of one's own worth, and to be freed of the burden of guilt. Even patients who strive toward a dominant goal will shun any activity that does not eventually lead toward their overriding objective. Any involvement that is simply fun is carefully avoided because it induces guilt or shame.

A general characteristic of all types of depression-prone individuals which is apparent throughout their lives and not only during clinical episodes is an almost paranoid feeling that others are overly conscious of their behavior. They uniformly see themselves as the center of other people's attention and thus pursue what they believe is model behavior. This characteristic is closely linked with the fear of autonomous gratification in that such individuals can never actively have fun because they are sure that others will deem them foolish or wasteful. Such individuals live highly restricted and hypermoral lives, not from any superior inner ethical code, but because they feel themselves to be constantly observed by others. These individuals also tend to be obsessive and to find safety in conformity and rituals. They constantly speak about one's duty and obligations and are quick to point out the trivial failings of others in a superior, haughty manner. In actuality, these individuals who go by the book often make life miserable for those around them, reproaching them for not living up to some imagined set of standards and constantly accusing those close to them of having humiliated them in public.

In therapy such individuals reveal that as children they were constantly observed by overly critical parents who expected model behavior from them in order to bring honor or acceptance to the family. As described by Cohen et al. (1954), the childhood behavior of some future depressives was exploited by the parents in the search for upward social mobility. Such individuals soon learn to see their behavior as the constant object of public and parental attention. They also do to their children what had been done to them. As therapy progresses, they often reveal a secret desire to be just the opposite of what they pretend to be. All sorts of sexual, antisocial, and romantic desires emerge which had been strongly suppressed for fear of criticism from parents and later from society at large.

This fear of autonomous gratification appears to play a very significant role in depression and may be primarily responsible for the eventual precipitation of a clinical depressive episode that does not involve an environmental loss. Some depressives decompensate when they realize after years of self-deprivation that they will not receive some special reward which they believed would be granted to them. Others become depressed as a result of the joyless life that they have imposed on themselves; they gain no pleasure from life and yet feel unable to alter their way of living. One woman who presented a variety of psychosomatic complaints gradually became depressed when she saw herself trapped in an ungratifying mode of existence. She described her life as going through the motions of the role of an upper-class suburban wife and mother. She admitted that she detested her fundraising activities, her husband's business associates, her clubs, and the usual daily routine to which she nevertheless strictly adhered. Her feeling of being trapped in an apparently successful and enviable life had been the prevalent mode of seeing herself for many years. She had grown up in a wealthy mid-western suburb, but due to the Depression her family had lost most of their capital. However, they continued to live as if they were wealthy, though everyone knew they could not really afford their lifestyle. The parents insisted on carrying out this economic sham and were careful to instruct their children on proper behavior, pointing out to them that others would be observing them to see if their loss of wealth had affected their "breeding." Throughout her life this woman made choices that would ensure social approval at the expense of personal satisfaction. When she reached middle age, she began to realize that it was too late to do the things she had really wanted to do. She confessed that even if she had been younger she could not have allowed herself to go against a harsh code of conformity which she expected from herself, even though it brought her only misery, Her anger at having to live according to her self-imposed restrictions seemed to result in violent headaches, and her fear that she might act out her secret desires accounted for other bodily symptoms. Her current life, dismal as it seemed to her, at least offered a structured and secure code of behavior.

Without it she believed that she would feel not only sinful but alone, abandoned, and without a set course to follow.

Other patients could be presented who throughout their lives have always made the same, if ungratifying, choices. These choices appear to be predicated on the original dictates of the dominant parent and on the later transference of parental authority to current life relationships. Such individuals distort others to fill the role of the demanding, critical parent and then act according to these transferential distortions, culminating in an existence which does not allow pleasure and predisposes them to chronic depression with definite paranoid and obsessive features.

Bargain Relationship

Implicit in the depressive's dependency and inhibition is what may be called the bargain relationship, which typifies some depressives' mode of interpersonal relations. The bargain is simply that the depressive will deny himself autonomous satisfaction in return for nurturance from the dominant other. This relationship is initiated by the parent, but the depressive reestablishes it on unwitting transference objects. This *quid pro quo* relationship ensures that gratification and acceptance will be forthcoming if willingness for self-sacrifice is properly demonstrated.

This pathological mode of relating was hinted at by Cohen et al. in their study of manicdepressives (1954). They mentioned the patient's use of splitting a significant other into an all-good partial object and repressing the other's bad characteristics in order to idealize the important other. This other has to be inflated and seen as totally good so that the patient can then depend on and utilize the other for his own needs. Jacobson also implied a similar relationship, employing orthodox terminology: "The libidinal cathexis of their selfrepresentations thus depends on the maintenance of a continuous libidinal hypercathexis of the love object, designed to prevent its aggressive devaluation in which their self is bound to participate" (1971, p. 259). Therefore, according to Jacobson the depressive must idealize the dominant other if he is to prevent a devaluation of the self which would precipitate a depressive episode. Actually, in some cases the other may be overvalued so that he can give structure to the depressive. In other cases the dominant other is utilized to absolve guilt, and in still other cases he is needed as a source of constant applause and selfless love.

An example of the first type of bargain relationship, in which structure is given by the significant other, is a brilliant graduate student who did extremely well under the tutelage of his professor. The student had a godlike reverence for the senior man and would consult him about all of his life decisions. He felt himself to be safe and secure as long as the professor approved of his work, and he subtly used the older colleague to structure his day and to plan his lectures and research. While he was fawning in regard to the professor, this student was indifferent to his wife, competitive and suspicious with his fellow students, and generally terrified of life outside the university. However, he managed well until the time came to do his dissertation. His professor found the student a prestigious job in a physics think tank where he could support himself while doing his thesis. The young man took the job without questioning his elder's choice, though it entailed moving to a nearby suburb and essentially cutting himself off from all regular contact with the university.

In his new job the student felt immediately uncomfortable; there was no academic hierarchy, people did their own jobs without competing, and the atmosphere was loose and egalitarian. Worst of all, the director of the institute was a quiet and benevolent figure who did not interfere in the lives of his employees, all of whom were expected to be mature selfdirected scientists. The student gradually became depressed in these new surroundings. He could not work unless he felt he was being observed and supervised by an esteemed superior, and the director simply refused to take on the role that the former professor had filled. Without the secure sense that a dominant other was watching and directing him, this promising scientist lost all interest in physics. He began to bother his co-workers with elementary questions in order to gain attention and developed a great dislike for the director for not fulfilling his inappropriate needs. When he was deprived of the structure supplied by the dominant other, all activities became meaningless. The student gradually started staying in bed, complaining to his wife, and having difficulty sleeping. His dreams of being empty and lost reflected his waking psychological state.

In this case the positive or gratifying aspects of the bargain relationship are illustrated rather than the more painful type of bond in which coercion by guilt is prominent and usually results in a more severe form of depression. In the latter case, the dominant other is needed to reassure against feelings of inherent evil and badness. In addition to an air of helpless resignation and a sense of worthlessness, these patients believe themselves to be inordinately vile and malicious and they are convinced that only the dominant other can free them this selfimage. One such patient who required brief hospitalization described herself in the most derogatory terms imaginable, whereas in reality she seemed to have led an exemplary life. Her mother was a selfish woman who resented any responsibility and detested the mothering role. When her husband left her, she blamed the patient and repeatedly told her that if she had never been born the father would have remained. The mother continued to blame her for her later misfortunes and in addition projected all sorts of sexual desires onto the patient, eventually making her believe that her incestuous desires had driven her father from the house. This woman accepted the blame for her mother's unhappiness and dedicated her life to seeking forgiveness. She could not tolerate her mother's being cross or angry, and she did everything she could to soothe or please her. For more than twenty years this woman forced her husband and children to visit the mother weekly in another city where the patient would fuss over her and try to win her praise. The patient's mood for the following week depended on the success of these Sunday outings.

This woman became severely depressed when she developed intimate feelings for her employer. She could not tolerate her desires, which proved to her that her mother had been right in the estimation that she was wanton and base. All her previous efforts to redeem herself were now without meaning. She would never change; she had always been and always would be evil and worthless. She succumbed to the image of herself that she despised and which disgusted her.

A third example of the bargain relationship can be illustrated by a businessman who demanded to be adulated and nurtured by his wife. However, his needs appeared insatiable; he had to be told constantly that he was loved and that he was appreciated. If the wife dared to express interest in any topic that did not concern him, he would become hurt and begin to pout or to berate his wife for not realizing how hard he worked for her welfare. At times he would threaten to leave her just so she could beg him to stay. On the rare occasions when his wife told him that she felt "sucked dry" by his demands, he punished her by crying and going through his speech of being unappreciated. The wife eventually unconsciously evolved her own defensive maneuvers by developing (and on occasion feigning) illness so that he could not ask her for nurturance.

This man feared that his wife would abandon him at any moment and his manipulations were pathological attempts to continue his needed relationship with her. At times he was also convinced that he was unlovable and so had to put his wife to the test to see if she really loved him, which meant he was worthy of love. While his behavior might appear controlling and even sadistic, as Rado (1928) described the depressive and his love object, this man truly believed that he was only trying to get the love he so desperately desired. His pathological needs blinded him to the destructive effect he had on his spouse. When she was sick and therefore not in danger of leaving him, he became solicitous and kind, only to revert again when she appeared healthy. This man had a long history of depressions following emotional abandonments throughout his life. He had married a submissive and frightened women in order to ensure that she would stay with him, and he continued to fight off his neurotic fear of abandonment by his machinations. It must be mentioned that her effect on him was totally out of proportion: if she smiled and told him she loved him at breakfast, he felt sure of himself the entire day; if she were sleepy and quiet, he felt depressed and neglected.

This bargain relationship demonstrates the depressive's excessive reliance on a dominant other for maintenance of self-worth and a sense of meaning. It may take various forms, but basically it is a revival of a real or fantasied childhood relationship in which the parent was able to grant the child a needed state of self in return for appropriate behavior.

Finally it should be stressed that what predisposes one to depression in the bargain relationship is not only the exclusivity but also the quality of the relationship. For example,

Lewinsohn (1969) suggested that depressives tend to limit their range of personal interactions. This conclusion seems valid but incomplete. An individual may lead a happy, productive life with only a few mutual, sharing relationships and not become depressed upon termination of these relationships. It is only when the relationship serves pathological needs, prevents autonomous gratification, and enforces the inhibition of independent self-worth that a predisposition to depression exists.

Felt Helplessness To Alter The Environment

As a result of this excessive reliance on external agents for gratification, and in certain cases for structure, the depressive displays a glaring lack of mastery over self-rewarding functions. Some are so constricted by strong inhibitions that they simply cannot overcome the guilt and shame that accompanies simple enjoyment. Every act that might be perceived as pleasurable must be rationalized and disguised as leading to a productive or serious goal. These individuals experience intense anxiety at even the dim prospect of enjoyment, so that they strongly shun such activities. Therefore they complain that they are helpless to alter their depression and they feel overwhelmed and weak. Other depressed individuals who depended on a dominant other for gratification feel similarly hopeless and helpless if this other is lost. However, these individuals are not really helpless but they would rather be depressed than break the taboos that they impose on themselves. Obviously this is not true of all depressed states: some people face situations which they are indeed helpless to alter. However, these individuals usually do not totally collapse in their efforts; they may feel frustrated, cheated, and angry, but not uniformly depressed. In addition, nondepressives do not display the undue emphasis on moral issues which are so often seen in individuals with recurrent depressions who must see everything as someone's fault—usually their own. Healthier individuals also do not show the characteristic maneuvers of involving others to relieve their suffering through manipulation and guiltinducing behavior that is seen in neurotic depression. To repeat what Sandler and Joffe (1965) elaborated in detail: we are all susceptible to the initial psychobiological response of depression which carries with it a transient sense of helplessness, but only selected individuals will progress to a clinical episode of depression in which the sense of helplessness is magnified and utilized to control others to reinstate the lost sense of well-being.

Seligman (as mentioned in chapter 2) proposed a theory of learned helplessness to account for some forms of depression. Seligman essentially postulated that the depression-prone individual has learned that action does not result in reinforcement of needs, and so he gives up and gradually lapses into a state of depression. Actually, the depressive is far from helpless in that he is adept at manipulating others and also is capable of impressive accomplishments when required to gain love or approval. Rather, the depressive's apparent helplessness results from a disruption in his usual mode of behaving and gaining esteem through pathological means. The sense of helplessness is both an automatic and pathological attempt to induce others to supply the needed reassurance, and it is a result of training that one must act in reaction to others in order to win the desired acknowledgment. Therefore learned helplessness does account for some aspects of depression, but it is limited to the areas of assertion and pleasure without guilt or shame. It is understandable how the depressive might superficially appear to demonstrate that effort and reward are unrelated, yet on closer inspection it becomes evident that his efforts are just more surreptitious and devious in achieving their reinforcements.

Two depressed patients will be briefly described who had an overwhelming sense of helplessness. It is of interest that while both had histories of only mild depression, both had received electroconvulsive therapy (which effected only temporary relief). Their air of helplessness may have resulted in their being given this form of treatment since they refused to take any responsibility for their own therapy once they became depressed. In retrospect, they appeared to derive some pleasure out of being thought of by loved ones as severely incapacitated and requiring hospital care and shock treatment.

One of these patients was a woman of thirty-five who had suffered her first depressive episode fifteen years earlier when she was in college. Her mother was a teacher and had essentially ordered the patient to attend a local teacher's college while continuing to live at home. Throughout her childhood this woman had been trained to gauge her own worth by the amount of approval she received from her mother. She was restricted from playing with others and her nonscholastic pursuits were severely criticized. However, she was allowed— indeed strongly encouraged—to achieve in school. This woman remembered that as a child whenever she excelled in some scholastic activity, she would immediately think of her mother and hoped that the latter would be pleased. The woman's father was a pleasant but weak figure in the household. His role was to earn money (which was never enough for the mother) and to appease his wife. Another clear message that the mother gave to the patient was that the world was a very dangerous place where others would trick you and take advantage of you. The mother further implied that the patient was no match for such a world and could only survive with the mother's protection.

As the patient reached adolescence, she began to rebel mildly against the mother, mostly in her fantasies. Boys started to show an interest in her and she was starting to derive pleasure outside the maternal orbit. She made secret plans to leave her local teacher's college and to go to an out-of-town university where she could live on her own and study what she herself chose. At this point her father suffered a severe heart attack which necessitated giving up his job. As a result, they shortly experienced financial problems and her hopes of leaving home were thwarted. With their dwindling income the mother became even more critical of the father, whom she berated in the crudest terms. The patient found it impossible to live at home with her mother, who appeared to have been continually angry, yet she did not see how she could afford to live on her own. Her one escape was to marry a young local businessman who did not fit her romantic ideal although he did offer a haven from the unhappy situation at home.

These were the circumstances in which she suffered her first attack of depression. The reasons for her decompensation appear fairly clear. She could no longer please her mother, who had become obsessed with money and filled with venom against the world. Furthermore, the mother had changed in the patient's own eyes; the patient now saw her as uniformly punishing and abusive. The patient wanted to defend her father who, after all, had supported the household until his illness, but she dared not assert herself against the mother. She also was not assertive or adventurous enough to move out on her own and support herself. Instead she chose the security of a marriage which rapidly revealed that it would not satisfy her needs.

After recovering from her initial depression she returned to school, received her teaching degree, and from then on felt herself locked in a profession and a marital union which were both ungratifying. Her husband furthered her sense of helplessness by discouraging any social or personal activities that she might independently enjoy. Throughout the remainder of her life and until she entered psychotherapy, she succumbed to a semiparasitic and largely childish existence. Whenever external pressures, such as having a child, put additional demands on her, she became depressed.

It is noteworthy that in her dreams during therapy, she repeatedly returned to the original situation in college. Another telling incident about this patient was that as she began showing signs of assertion, her husband tried to get her to discontinue therapy in spite of her history of frequent hospitalizations. It is to her credit that she refused his demands and decided to pay for her therapy herself. At the beginning of her therapy, this woman exuded a sense of helplessness, of everything being too much trouble, of being incapable of any independent action. She wanted things done for her, and to be taken care of by others or to be told what to do by others. She did not dare to make any decisions on her own. However, she had been far from helpless in other areas; she was a competent teacher, housewife, and mother. Her area of helplessness centered on assertion of her beliefs and independence from the evaluations of others.

The second patient was in his late twenties but already had been given two courses of electroconvulsive therapy. Initially, he constantly complained of being ineffectual and of being mistreated by others. Actually, he was very adept at indirectly getting his own way by manipulating those around him. He never considered the numerous times when other people tried to help him or treated him fairly. He focused only on those incidents when others had not lived up to his own idiosyncratic code of honor and had not accorded him special treatment. His two depressions had occurred when he could not get what he wanted, namely, the approval or special attention from esteemed others through his usual machinations. This patient believed he was helpless, but what actually occurred was that his usual mode of controlling others had failed.

This young man had been raised in an atmosphere of deception, secret deals, and obligating behavior and he could not at first consider any other mode of conduct. This form of interaction had become automatic and unconscious. What remained in consciousness was a highly exaggerated response to the slightest rebuff and a feeling that everyone should go out of their way for him. The following excerpt is from a note he brought to one of his early sessions in order to convey his plight:

> My heart is so affected by things, it cries. I am sad and I can't stop it and say "be happy." It just doesn't seem to do any good. But what else can I do— do it myself or have it done for me. What can I do. Something has to be done before one day I jump off a bridge or at least seriously want to. Will it pass? I pray, but if God exists I don't even know if he cares —look at the world we live in. I am lost.

On the surface, this pathetic passage may illustrate the helplessness this patient felt in terms of improving his condition; others had to do it for him. However, during the time he wrote this passage he reluctantly worked at his job and even gloated over making some especially good business deals. His despair actually related to being unable to attain the special recognition he felt he deserved from his father, who was also his boss.

There is no doubt that even mild depression can be an incapacitating illness which not only involves a felt sense of helplessness but also may affect an individual's level of performance. However, when the origin of this feeling of helplessness is traced psychotherapeutically what usually emerges is that the individual first felt helpless in achieving meaning or gratification either as praise from a dominant other or in pursuit of a dominant goal. Having failed in these pursuits, the individual finds little meaning in any of life's other activities and his sense of helplessness generalizes to his entire social space. In other depressed individuals, such as the woman just described, the individual has made choices throughout life that lock him into an ungratifying existence. Here again the individual lacks the courage to break his self-imposed taboos and thus despairs of his helplessness first to gain pleasure and eventually to accomplish even the most rudimentary tasks.

The Cognitive Avoidance of Overt Anger

In a recent paper on depression, Coyne (1976) related a strange cure for depression practiced by a Dr. Williams of London in the early nineteenth century. When a depressed individual consulted Dr. Williams, he informed the patient that he should seek out a certain doctor in Scotland who was famous for his ability to cure the disorder. The patient obediently journeyed to Scotland only to find that the highly able physician did not exist. After this fruitless search, the patient found that "a desire to upbraid (Dr. Williams) had engaged his entire thoughts on his way home, to the complete exclusion of his original complaint cited" (Coyne, 1976, p. 38). This anecdote suggests what has been almost universally found by authors on depression: the affect of depression is incompatible with the overt expression of anger. This finding has led to specific behavior modification techniques (although less circuitous than those of Dr. Williams) to evoke anger in depressed patients by assigning them to monotonous, repetitive, and ungratifying tasks until the patient "blows up" and anger replaces depression (Taulbee and Wright, 1971). On the other hand, the incompatibility of overt anger and depression has also led to the notion that depression is a result of repressed rage. Indeed, as described in chapter 2, some have seen it as misdirected anger which torments the ego or the self-image.

The fact that clinical depression appears to decrease as the ability to directly express anger is displayed, however, does not prove this "repressed rage" hypothesis. Brenner (1975) reviewed a number of contributions which assert that enjoyment is also incompatible with the affect of depression. Does this prove then that enjoyment is repressed during depression and therapy should induce the patient to "get the enjoyment out"? It gradually becomes evident that direct repression of an affect is a complicated affair, if such a process can occur at all. What actually appears to be the case is that an individual's unconscious cognitive system structures a situation to produce a specific effect. Therefore the depressive does not overtly display anger because he automatically structures his view of himself and others so that anger is not produced. Rather, the depressive appears to respond to what most individuals call anger-producing situations with self-blame, feelings of hurt, or some sort of excusing the other. Rather than simply assuming that the depressive represses anger or directs it at himself, a search for the cognitive distortions which fail to elicit an aggressive response may be more productive.

The depressive's lack of overt anger recently has been interpreted in terms of his tenuous object relations. The expression of anger may antagonize the dominant other and jeopardize the depressive's sources of gratification. For example, Arieti (1974) described that anger in depressives ultimately leads to more depression; it creates the fear that the dominant other will abandon the individual, which leads to an increased sense of loss and hopelessness. Anger is seen as a highly dangerous affect which must be concealed and suppressed. Klein's classic formulation of the depressive position emphasizes the infant's fear of losing his inner good objects through his aggressive wishes. She interpreted the infant as attributing the pain and frustration of loss to his own angry behavior with a subsequent suppression of overt hostility. If Klein's basic formulations are extended to the interpersonal sphere, the depressives plight of being angry while in a state of need for nurturance from the other, and the resultant fear of the manifestation of that anger, becomes more understandable. To express anger directly means to lose the allimportant other who supplies the incorporated good objects, that is, gratification and selfesteem. The depressive eventually believes that any expression of anger will catastrophically result in the loss of gratification.

The depressive's lack of overt hostility can also be due to his distortion of relationships. Some depressives idealize the dominant other and so implicitly trust the other's judgment that they see no reason for resentment or anger. If they fail to obtain the other's acceptance, it is because they have not tried hard enough to be worthy, and not because the other is stingy or unjust. They feel they have only themselves to blame and thus have no cause to become angry. A middle-aged depressed woman, describing the failure of her considerable attempts to win praise and love from her father, exclaimed, "What is wrong with me that he doesn't love me?" This woman could not conceive of her father as ungiving or unloving; it was her fault that she could not please him. Although married and the mother of three children, she still believed that her chief role in life was to please her father and devote herself to him. As in her childhood, her father was the only one who could make her happy and give meaning to her life. To alter her view of her father would have required an alteration of her entire mode of being.

Another possible reason for the depressive's inability to express anger is that the capacity to feel angry and to use anger as a direct mode of achieving an objective implies a sense of autonomy and independence that is just the ability the depressive lacks. These individuals are tuned to the reactions of others rather than to the expression of self, regardless of consequences. To become angry means to satisfy one's impulse without considering the effect on others, and it requires exactly the sense of self that the depressive has not developed. Thus he resorts to more reliable manifestations of displeasure such as pouting or suffering, which produce the appropriate impact on others—guilt and forgiveness. Some depressives that Bonime (1967) so aptly described are stubbornly uncooperative in therapy; they spitefully refuse to take their share of responsibility and take pride in their resistance to change. Manipulation and control of others seem to be the cardinal features of their activity. This type of depressive, which is similar to Arieti's claiming type, may be understood as rebelling against the disappointments in past bargain relationships. These individuals feel themselves cheated by past dominant others who did not fulfill their promise, real or imagined, in return for selfsacrifice. These patients then resolve never to show any signs of true mutuality or cooperation as a way of punishing the dominant other, whose role the therapist has transferentially assumed. They will demand all sorts of favoritism and support while refusing to take any initiative in therapy and ultimately want to frustrate the therapist by not becoming what they believe he would wish them to be.

However, such patients never show anger overtly but punish the therapist by continually reminding him of their lack of improvement in therapy —that is, of the therapist's inability to change them. In this manner they make the therapist feel powerless and frustrated, but never give him cause to terminate the relationship. Thus they defeat the dominant other without losing him. Yet these patients continue to center their existence around the therapist and in reality defeat themselves in order allegedly to control the other. Their activity continues to be judged in terms of the effect it will have on the therapist and the reaction it will elicit. Living in a world of reflective gratification, the depressive cannot conceive of himself as acting simply for himself. His every thought and act implicates the other and includes the other's reaction.

A talented college student who began experiencing episodes of anxiety and depression as she approached graduation described this type of other-dependent relatedness. She became immediately attracted to any man who showed her attention and would rush into a close relationship without adequately evaluating the other person. Her main concern was that he be pleased with her, and she devoted herself to fitting into her boyfriends' preferences. Despite her efforts to hold onto the relationship and placate the other, she was often exploited and treated with little consideration. When this occurred, she persistently blamed herself for having been rejected. She believed that she had somehow offended the other or that she had not been sufficiently perceptive of the other's needs. The other was right even in mistreating her. Each failure to maintain a relationship proved to her that she would be an old maid and condemned to a life of solitude. She believed that the only way she might escape abandonment would be to surrender autonomy and spontaneity. Any display of assertiveness, especially of anger or disagreement, would surely drive the other away. This young woman did occasionally get angry, but always after the fact: in the presence of esteemed others, she was overcome with the desire to please and to endear herself. Even her considerable gifts were at the mercy of others, and a project that had taken her months to prepare became worthless if mildy criticized by a teacher. The teacher's judgment was never in question: if she had only worked harder, she might have pleased him.

A specific confirmation of the lack of repressed anger in mildly depressed patients comes from studies of their dreams. If they were bursting with unexpressed rage rather than distorting their view of the world in order to avoid anger, their dreams should reveal the repressed hostility. Beck and his colleagues examined the dreams of 218 patients who were independently rated by two judges as nondepressed, moderately depressed, and severely depressed. The major characteristics of the dreams of the depressed groups was a consistent masochistic trend. The dreams of the depressed patients revealed themes of disappointment, rejection, humiliation, or other similar unpleasant experiences, but the dreams did not exhibit notable anger.

Hauri (1976) reviewed some of the literature on the dreams of depressed patients as well as reporting his own study on eleven patients remitted from depression and who were matched with eleven control subjects. Past studies had shown that several depressed individuals report dreams that are bland, barren, and involve mainly family members. As depression lifts the dreams become more conflictual, although masochistic and dependency themes persist even after clinical improvement.

Hauri's own study is noteworthy in that patients who had recovered from a depressive episode were selected and therefore their dreams reflected basic personality structure rather than the possible distortions of an acute depressive state. In addition, Hauri utilized allnight EEG tracings and awakened each subject to report dreams in order to reduce selective recall of only pleasant or socially acceptable dreams. In comparing recovered depressives with control subjects, Hauri found a number of significant differences in their dreams. Dreams of remitted depressive patients showed more past than present or future events, more unhappy than happy emotions, and more action exerted by nonhuman entities (storms, motors, bullets, and so on). Equally important was the finding that depressives did not show more hostility toward others or hostility toward the self in the dreams. Hauri commented that this may be the most important result of his study. Hauri concluded that on the basis of dream content, the depressive may see the world as dangerous or ungiving or even hostile, but this hostility neither emanates from the dreamer nor is directed against him.

Even Bonime, who believes that much neurotic depressive behavior is a distorted manifestation of anger, does not report excessive aggression in the dreams of depressed patients presented in his book, *The Clinical Use of Dreams* (1968). His work as well as that of Beck does not support the repressed rage hypothesis.

Overt anger may occasionally be seen in some mildly depressed individuals when they view their situation more realistically. This may occur through therapeutic effort, or in some individuals before change through treatment. They can experience periods of insight when they are not blinded by their needs and distortions. This is usually not the case with severe depressives for whom reality has become completely transformed in its meaning. However, even in mildly depressed patients these periods are short-lived and the patients return to their accustomed mode of cognitive interpretation of events.

On the few occasions that I have observed depressive openly express anger, their expression was consistently clothed in moralistic terms with great attempts to justify the outburst. Even then the show of anger was not a simple expression of self, but a calculated attempt to coerce another to do something or to justify the feeling of depression by showing how they had been mistreated. Cohen and her co-workers (1954) also were not impressed with the importance of anger in their study of manicdepressive patients. The conclusions they reached are:

> We have said little in this report about the manic-depressive's hostility. We feel that it

has been considerably over-stressed as a dynamic factor in the illness. Certainly, a great deal of the patient's behavior leaves a hostile impression upon those around him, but we feel that the driving motivation in the patient is the one we have stressed—the feeling of need and emptiness. The hostility we would relegate to a secondary position; we see hostile feelings arising in the patient as the result of frustration of his manipulative and exploitative needs. We conceive of such subsequent behavior—demandingness toward the other or selfinjury—as being an attempt to restore the previous dependent situation (1954, p. 252).

The Washington group further adds "that much of the hostility that has been imputed to the patient has been the result of his annoying impact on others rather than of a primary motivation to do injury to them."

Perhaps much of the confusion of the role of anger in depressed states owes its origin to differences of opinion regarding both the nature of depression and of anger. As Mendelson (1974) accurately observed, there is no uniform consensus about the definition of either affect. Some psychoanalysts require the presence of aggression in some form or other as necessary for the diagnosis of depression. These manifestations can be self-recriminations (selfdirected anger), low self-esteem (aggressive cathexis of the self-representation), or manipulativeness (controlling others by anger). This difference of opinion shows the equal lack of agreement on the nature of aggression. When Jacobson writes about an aggressive cathexis, she is describing a highly abstract metapsychological process that does not coincide with the overt, conscious expression of anger as known to the layman. The same is true of the intersystemic conflict between ego and superego. However, Bonime (1960) conceives of aggression as the covert motive of the depressive's behavior in his lack of cooperation in therapy or his control of others. Here aggression is implied from nonaggressive behavior by its end result or by its alleged motive. Still other psychiatrists describe anger or aggression as a felt state of self—of being angry. Therefore it appears that there is a discrepancy in the psychiatric literature as to whether aggression should be seen as a primary instinct or form of psychic energy (that cannot by definition be directly experienced), as a motive force behind behavior which is not phenomenologically felt as anger, or as a primary feeling state.

Despite this confusion over the conceptual status of aggression, it is clinically evident that the depressive shuns the direct expression and even the experience of anger. He does not use overt anger in the service of his needs; rather, he utilizes manipulativeness to control others. If this manipulativeness is termed a form of anger or aggression, then this special use of the term should be made explicit.

The extreme emphasis on the role of hostility in depression may be a lingering influence of Freud's original theories stated in *Mourning and Melancholia,* which described a good deal of depressive symptomatology as misdirected aggression. As Mendelson (1974) wisely observed: "Freud's explanation of the melancholic's self-reproaches and Abraham's description of the manic-depressive's ambivalence became universally and, it is feared, uncritically and uniformly applied to all depressive phenomena. And later authors frequently sought to justify these constructions rather than to investigate their applicability" (p. 194).

Family Background of Mild Depressives

As mentioned in chapter 2, there is a paucity of studies on family transactions in depression as compared with schizophrenia. The few studies that have attempted to determine the childhood roots of adult depression mainly have centered on the experience of parental loss. This interest in childhood bereavement appears stimulated by the hypotheses that adult depression is the reawakening of a childhood trauma, or that object loss is the basic problem in depressive disorders. Most studies have compared the frequency of the death of a parent during the childhood years of adult depressed patients and of matched controls. The results of these studies have been contradictory except for the finding that childhood loss (through death of a parent, divorce, or some other form of separation) is more common in all forms of psychiatric disorders, especially delinquency. Brown (1968) made an additional intriguing observation: 55 percent of the poets listed in the *Oxford Book of English Verse* and the *Dictionary of National Biography* (in England) lost a father or mother before the age of fifteen. This is a higher rate of parental death than is found in depressive (or delinquent) samples. Brown speculated that these poets turned to internal sources of gratification through fantasy to soften the blow of the parental loss, and their native genius later allowed these fantasies to be expressed poetically.

The rate of parental loss may not be the significant factor for later disturbance if it is taken in isolation. The effect of the loss on the surviving parent, the subsequent disruption of the family, the availability of substitutes, the child's age at the time of the loss, and his conception of the loss must all be taken into account in retrospective studies. Loss of a parent through death or other misfortune is certainly a significant childhood trauma but it does not appear specifically to predispose one to depression as an adult. To view the adult depressive as the recapitulation of an actual childhood loss is somewhat simplistic. Freud, who originated this concept of reactivated childhood trauma, did not intend the actual loss of the parent but the loss of the parent's love, which is a totally different matter.

This loss of love may then represent an unconscious decathexis of the object representation and thus an unconscious object loss, but it is not meant to imply a loss of the parent in reality. Here again a metapsychological hypothesis and clinical data become confused. Sandler and Joffe (1965) tried to clarify the matter by stressing that depression is not the result of the loss of an object but a state of well-being of the self supplied by the object.

Cohen et al. (1954) did attempt a retrospective reconstruction of the childhoods of their twelve manic-depressive cases. They did not find evidence of early object loss or of a childhood depressive reaction equivalent to Abraham's "primal parathymia" (1924). Rather, these investigators noted that the families felt isolated or ostracized from the mainstream of society, the mothers blamed the fathers for the alleged social failure, and the child was expected to redeem the family's honor or prestige. In terms of more specific child rearing, this group found that the mother accepted the child when he was a helpless infant but began to reject him when he displayed the normal willfulness of a toddler. These findings are confirmed by Arieti in chapter 6: in the early childhood of severe depressives the mother is initially giving and loving but quickly begins to make stringent demands on the child so that continued nurturance is contingent on the child's fulfillment of expectations. The important aspect of this interpersonal relationship for the child is the realization that love can be abruptly withdrawn if parental expectations are not met.

It may not be an actual loss that predisposes the individual to depression, but the constant fear that a loss can occur if the proper behavior is not forthcoming.

A later development noted both by Cohen et al. (1954) and Arieti is that the parent assumes the power to redeem the child, to make him feel worthy. The child is convinced that it is his own fault if he does not achieve this redemption: if he had tried harder he could have obtained the needed support of the parent. This interchange sets up the process by which the adult depressive attempts to attain love by obedience and hard work, blaming himself if he does not achieve his objective. Much of this aspect of the future depressive already has been covered in chapter 6 and will not be repeated here. It is sufficient to note that the child's failure to fulfill parental expectations is experienced as guilt and worthlessness.

Slipp (1976) studied the family setting that produces a depressive individual. He found that the child is given a contradictory message from the parents: the child is expected to succeed socially and at the same time expected to fail, so as not to become too independent of the parents.

Slipp described the parents as expecting achievement and yet simultaneously rewarding failure. The child learns to succeed but fears that this success will bring abandonment. According to Slipp:

> The depressive evolves an oppositional form of symbiosis as a compromise solution to this double bind. By partial compliance to both succeed and fail messages, he does not risk abandonment by either parent; yet by rebelling sufficiently against these injunctives, he preserves some autonomy. Through halfhearted performances to his parents' wishes, he can play off both pressures and avoid being either strong or totally helpless. By partially defeating himself and losing he can claim to be a victim of external circumstances, and he does not have to take responsibility (1976, p. 398).

Therefore Slipp traces the pathological behavior of the adult depressive to the childhood solution of a double message: succeed for the family but fail lest you become independent of the family.

While I do not agree with every aspect of Slipp's analysis, the observations presented by him are important in demonstrating how the experience of independent success is perverted in the childhood of future depressives. In my experience, some future depressives have been given a clear message to succeed, but the success later was robbed of its meaning; rather, it was presented as rightful repayment to the parent, as simply keeping up with the alleged superiority of the family, or as a way to get love from the parent. The child was told to succeed but that he should not enjoy his success.

The disparities between the childhoods of severe and mild depressives appear to be more a function of the amount of this thwarting of development than a function of qualitative differences. As a rule, the childhood of mild depressives was not so blunted by moralistic blaming and early threats of abandonment. Often the patients were made to feel weak or lazy rather than evil. They also did not have to work as hard or to distort their perceptions as much to gain parental approval. They often were the family favorites and were able to maintain this role by compliance. Therefore their inducements for buying the parental distortions were positive (favoritism, praise) rather than negative (guilty recriminations, threats of abandonment). Finally, for most but not all mild depressives, the father rather than the mother was the dominant parent. This finding was also reported by Slipp (1976). While such individuals soon became imbued with the family distortions that everyone owed everything to the father and their task was to insure the father's benevolence, they managed to continue a close relationship with a loving though weak and submissive mother. The threat of abandonment also came at a later stage of development and so had less impact on the personality. It was not until such individuals could bring social value to the family by model behavior or excellent grades that the father became interested in them. Before this time they were treated as unimportant charges of the mother.

Nevertheless, in these individuals as well as in the severe melancholics there is a basic instability of self-esteem. They also have been unable to internalize sources of worth and must constantly derive their meaning as individuals from external agencies. They remain forever excessively vulnerable to the disappointments and losses which, for better or worse, form part of human destiny.

Notes

[14] Some confirmatory evidence for considering depression (as a primary feeling state and not as a clinical syndrome) as a basic psychobiological response is that it can be produced by physiological means. Mild depressions can be observed following viral illnesses or in states of fatigue. Depression also can accompany hypothyrodism or pancreatic disease or be produced by drugs such as reserpine. All this seems

to indicate that depression, while most frequently caused by psychological events, is closely tied to basic neurochemical alterations and thus appears to be a fundamental mode of reaction which is similar to other emotions.

PSYCHODYNAMICS OF DEPRESSION AND SUICIDE IN CHILDREN AND ADOLESCENTS

Jules Bemporad

Chapter 4 was concerned with an exposition of the clinical syndromes of depressionlike disorders in children and adolescents. This chapter will attempt a deeper look at the phenomenon of childhood depression, going beyond clinical descriptions to theoretical issues.

For decades the classical psychoanalytic position on the possibility of depression in childhood was firm and unanimous: it could not exist. Rochlin (1959) plainly stated that depression, by definition, is a result of an inward deflection of aggression mediated by a strong superego. Since the superego does not exist in young children, neither could depression. Beres (1966) also expressed the belief that depression, as a primary superego phenomenon involving intersystemic conflict, must be manifested by predominant sustained guilt which is absent in children.

Even psychoanalysts who did not emphasize the older retroflected anger hypothesis of depression expressed grave doubts over the possibility of this affect or its development into the clinical syndrome before adolescence. Rie (1966) in an excellent review of the theoretical literature argues that even if depression is conceptualized as low self-esteem resulting from a discrepancy between the ego ideal and the actual self, there is great difficulty in applying this model to children. The difficulty is that a stable self-representation is not expected to develop, on theoretical grounds, until adolescence. Rie concludes, "Hence, the major dynamic elements of depression, perhaps not inappropriately regarded as the essence of depression, and indeed some of their structural antecedents, seem not to be generated in toto until the end of latency age" (p. 679). Mahler (1961) also sums up the matter quite unequivocally: "We know that the systematized affective disorders are unknown in childhood. It has been conclusively established that the immature personality structure of the infant or older child is not capable of producing a state of depression as that seen in the adult" (p. 342).

Despite this unanimity of distinguished opinion, depressionlike states do appear in children, theory notwithstanding. Mendelson (1974) has taken the theorists to task over their lack of clinical familiarity with the subject matter that they have so elegantly discussed and dismissed. He writes of the theoretical literature on childhood depression: "It would seem that in no other area of the psychoanalytic literature on depressives are the theoretical papers so far removed from the observations that any clinician can make in the course of his daily practice" (p. 165).

The conflict between theory and observation is far from new in the history of thought (Kuhn, 1962). When such a clash occurs, either the observations are in error or the theory needs revision. As documented in chapter 4, more clinicians are reporting depressionlike states in children; thus we must turn to the underlying theory in our search for error. Indeed, most of the authors who make the claim that depression in childhood is *a priori* impossible subscribe to the orthodox Freudian view of melancholia. If a different theoretical framework is adopted, then a more workable and harmonious interrelation between deduction and observation may evolve. What appears to be most sorely needed is a system of childhood development that stays within the general boundaries of psychoanalytic thought and modifies certain postulates to be more in line with clinical observations and experimental research. Unfortunately, much classical psychoanalytic thought has ignored findings from allied disciplines, and due to this insularity it has become limited in dealing with various clinical problems. The growth or true evaluation of any explanatory system appears to require a healthy interchange between observation and inference.

Even on a strictly theoretical level, the classical psychoanalytic formulations can be found wanting in certain considerations of the development of affect in children. There does not appear to be a sufficient acknowledgement of the gradual accretion of abilities or the gradual consolidation of internal psychic structures over a period of years. Even if the usefulness (one cannot say validity) of such concepts as the superego or the self-representation is agreed upon and accepted, the consolidation of these structures must be thought of as a very gradual process. However, a more evident failing of classical theory is its almost total disregard of cognitive factors in the affective development of the child. The ability to experience certain affects and the advancement of cognitive structures are intertwined development. As indicated throughout Piaget (1951) cognition and affect are but two aspects of the same evolving unity of the child's psyche.

Without the ability to cognitively appreciate certain aspects of experience, specific affects can not be experienced. Therefore a consideration of cognitive development must go hand in hand with any attempt to understand the development of affect. This does not necessarily mean that the processes of understanding that give rise to emotions must be conscious, any more than Piaget's cognitive schemata are explicitly conscious. Rather, these schemata are unconscious principles that organize experience and give the experience its meaning and thus its emotional content.

This concomitant aspect of cognitive and affective development has been described by Arieti (1967), who postulates that there are various levels of emotions which develop during ontogenesis. This view is founded on a good deal of theoretical logic as well as experimental evidence. Werner (1948) definitively showed that one of the major processes of development is differentiation. He conceived of the child as proceeding from a relatively global "syncretic" state to an articulated, differentiated mode of being. Therefore, the global positive experiences of the young infant gradually become separated into bodily pleasure, mastery, love, joy, or quiet satisfaction. Similarly, global negative experiences differentiate into the adult states of pain, fear, anxiety, depression, or despair. Although somewhat corrected by the recent developments of ego psychology, classical psychoanalysis has been guilty of a double error: ascribing an excessively precocious cognitive system to the child and an excessively immature motivational structure to adults. Just as young children cannot grasp the realities of the world as seen by the adult and therefore cannot experience the exact emotions of adults, mature individuals—by virtue of their developed cognitive state—are motivated by more highly differentiated feeling states than children. Experimental studies which partially support this view have been performed by Kohlberg (1969) in the area of moral development and by Loevinger (1976) in regard to overall ego development. These studies are extremely relevant to the study of the individual's affective experience at different stages of development, since they reveal a progression of the predominant modes of thought through ontogenesis. These studies have found that it is not until relatively late in childhood that the individual proceeds beyond a conformist point of view which simply accepts social rules without a great deal of self-awareness or freedom to reflect on multiple possibilities in situations. Loevinger states that many individuals never advance beyond this level and their inner life remains filled with banal clichès, shallow emotions, and simplistic moralizing. While it is possible that adults at this level of psychic development can experience depression, it appears certain that children who have not reached this level are incapable of depressed feelings, according to Loevinger's system.

Therefore, when conceptual systems other than classical psychoanalysis are considered, the question of depression in childhood becomes transformed. As stated in chapter 4, the problem is not whether adultlike depression can occur in childhood, but how the cognitive and affective limitations at different stages of childhood modify the experience and expression of emotions in general. Therefore the most fruitful approach to a theoretical discussion of childhood depression might begin from a developmental standpoint, although our current knowledge of the inner life of children is still very far from adequate. The implicit assumption in this discussion is that any affect necessitates the presence of unconscious cognitive structures which develop through childhood.

Another assumption is that depression is a direct affect much like anxiety (see Sandler and Joffe, 1965), free from complicated metapsychological events that are automatically experienced in certain situations by susceptible individuals. At the same time, depression is seen as a complex affect (see Arieti, 1967) which presupposes a good deal of cognitive maturation. Thus a more realistic search for the vicissitudes of depression would focus on ego development rather than the previous psychoanalytic emphasis on the evolution of the superego.

Depression and Development

Infancy

Syndromes which are phenomenologically comparable to adult depression have been described by Spitz (1946) and by Engel and Reichsman (1956). Spitz delineated the wellknown entity of "anaclitic depression" described in chapter 4. Engel and Reichsman reported a thirteen-month-old girl who withdrew into a state of sleep when strangers approached. From their observation of this young child, Engel and Reichsman postulated an innate "conservation withdrawal" reaction which they believed to be an infantile prototype of the "giving up" attitude in adult depression.

Although Spitz's observations included crying, withdrawal, and sad faces, he did not believe that this infantile behavior was the result of the same intrapsychic situation manifested by adult depressives, because the infants lacked the formation of a tyrannical superego which would direct aggressive drives toward the ego. However, Spitz speculated that self-directed aggression did play a role in these infants' symptoms since they lacked an external love object (the mother) who would both absorb the released aggression and stimulate the expression of libido, which would neutralize the aggression. Being deprived of a maternal figure, these infants directed their instinctual drives on themselves. In this manner Spitz appeared to maintain the concept of self-directed aggression as basic to depression while bypassing the theoretical problem that the infants had not yet formed a superego. However, even if Spitz's formulations are tentatively accepted, the problem remains as to who is the ultimate recipient of these aggressive drives. Jacobson (1971) postulates an aggressive cathexis of the self-representation in adult depression, but can we ascribe selfrepresentation to a six-month-old infant? Can we equally postulate a pathognomonic introject as the recipient of the aggression?

Herein lies the problem that arises when we consider Spitz's model of "anaclitic depression" as a form of depression at all. It appears that the young infant is simply too immature and his psyche too unformed actually to experience depression. There is certainly grave doubt whether infants of this age have any awareness of themselves, or what type of mentation actually exists. Piaget (1952) has in fact called the first eighteen to twenty-four months of life the sensory-motor stage, emphasizing his belief that at this early age mental life consists mainly of innate reactions, habit sequences, and possibly physical discomfort.

However, infants do appear distressed by separation from their mothers and after some time withdraw into a sort of detached, defensive state that Bowlby (1960) described. Thus there is a great temptation to ascribe feelings of depression to the infants' experiential state. This is a dangerous undertaking, for in so doing we may be projecting our own adult affects on the minds of infants. Anna Freud (1970) warned of this danger, writing that "some psychoanalysts credit the newborn already with complex mental processes, with a variety of affects which accompany the action of the various drives and, moreover, with complex reactions to these drives and actions, such as for instance guilt feelings."

We shall probably never exactly know what the infant who has been separated from his mother actually feels, but we can safely assume that he does not experience the same range or depth of emotion that are part of the adult's inner life. The abandoned infant has served as the prototype of adult depression, but such a relationship must be taken as metaphorical at best.

The dissimilarity between these infantile states and adult depression becomes more striking when we learn that lack of cognitive stimulation (Dennis and Najarian, 1957) or even malnutrition (Malmquist, 1971) can produce the same behavioral result. Yet these findings are not so surprising, since the mother serves the infant in countless ways. To use Piaget's terminology, she is the primary "ailment" for the infant's budding schemata. Her deprivation results in stunting psychic development, whether it is affective, cognitive, or motor. Probably all of these discrete functions may be syncretically intermeshed at this early age (Werner, 1948). Therefore loss of the mother may represent the same thing as losing stimulation or tangible nourishment. The mother allows the infant's mind to develop. Through her, the infant forms a sense of self and can begin to anchor himself in reality. The absence of proper mothering, because of its significant role in maturation, thus can result in such long-range deviations as described by Spitz and Bowlby. Early deprivation, if prolonged, does not lead to later depression, but to either retardation or psychopathy.

In this light, it might be more correct to

classify the reactions of the infant as development deprivations that are unpleasant but which may be as globally experienced by the immature psyche as persistent nonspecific pain or the absence of external stimulation. Since mental development may well begin with emotion and the infant may be capable of suffering long before it can think, there is no doubt that these states are painful, but there can be little relationship to the later pain of depression.

Even in later infancy, such as in the cases described by Engel and Reichsman (1956) and Bowlby (1960), it seems that turning away from the environment represents a possibly innate withdrawal reaction from an ungratifying world rather than true depression. In Bowlby's experience, after a period of time infants eventually will come out of their withdrawal and begin to interact with strangers.

Early Childhood

This developmental stage may be defined arbitrarily as beginning with the infant's psychological individuation from the mother. During this time there is a shift in the child's gratification processes; he now delights in actively doing rather than in being given to and passively nurtured (Mahler, 1968). This is the era of normal oppositionalism and the embryonic testing of the will. There is a delightful "love affair with the world," in which normal fears, apprehensions, or inhibitions are overruled by a constant curiosity about the external world. Clinical reports of depressionlike symptoms at this exuberant age are conspicuously absent. Yet this may be a crucial period for laying the initial groundwork of later depressive episodes.

At this stage the child appears to be faced with a critical choice: to satisfy his own pleasure in the exercise of his will and risk the censure of the parent, or to inhibit his spontaneity and insure the love of the parent. Silverberg (1952) has beautifully called this the conflict between the "heroic" and "unheroic" solution to childhood. Obviously, the eventual decision depends on the temperament of the child, the personality of the parent, the presence of siblings, the economic standard of the family, and an infinity of other factors. However, the initial battle between self-gratification and the surrender of the burgeoning self for the insurance of love leaves its scars long after the war is over. If the parent insists on perfect behavior or is threatened by the willfulness of the child, then a sense of self-inhibition will gradually crystallize and sow the seeds of later self-denial and fear of personal fulfillment. If there is as an additional complication a depressed parent who cannot participate in the joyous excitement of the child's discovery of the world, then a certain sense of deadness and lack of spontaneity may also evolve.

In retrospective studies, Cohen and her coworkers (1954) found that the mothers of later depressives were uncomfortable with their child's emergence from a passive infant into a willful toddler. Green (1946) in another context indicated that middle-class mothers create an exorbitant need for love in their children and then utilize the threat of withdrawal of love as a disciplinary measure. It may be just this form of sabotaging of the will not through physical punishment but through threats of abandonment or through shaming that causes the child to begin to associate free expression with loss of love or with causing harm in needed others. Mahler (1966) contended that the origins of a depressive mood state lie in the abrupt and simultaneous collapse of the young child's belief in his own omnipotence as well as that of his parents. This view also appears to ascribe psychological processes which are too sophisticated to the young child. Although the preschooler may act as if the world is his oyster and show an alarming lack of fear in dangerous situations, we cannot therefore assume that he believes himself (or others) to be omnipotent. Rather, the young child derives a primitive sense of pleasure in doing, what Freud termed *funktionlust* and Mahler herself described so well as part of the practicing subphase of the separation-individuation process. The roots of depression appear to reside in parental punishment and lack of response to the child's normal exploratory and mastery behavior, which leads to an automatic and unconscious inhibition of activities necessary for later development of an independent sense of worth through individual accomplishment.

Such children present a clinical picture of seriousness, a lack of spontaneity, and often a clinging relation to the parent. While displaying precocious self-control, they are immature in terms of venturing away from the needed parent. These children are being trained to inhibit and distrust their natural inclination toward mastery and autonomous gratification. They are already substituting their parent's pleasure for their own in order to continue the needed security of the parental relationship. To use Sullivanian terms, they are foregoing satisfaction needs for the insurance of security needs.

These children cannot be called depressed, although they may appear sad, frightened, and unduly serious. We do not know their feeling state; although they are able to verbalize, they cannot yet identify or describe emotions through language. We may diagnose these children as overly inhibited and at risk for later depression. Because they still inhabit an age-appropriate action world, they express their pathology through overt behavior. Even then they can alter their mood state readily as the situation demands. Thus if they are fortunate enough to attend a nursery school or be with adults who appreciate their spontaneity, they quickly become fun-loving active youngsters.

As Mahler (1966) aptly observed, they tend to show their symptoms in the presence of the parent, possibly because it is the parent who demands the submissive, controlled reaction. They do not as yet generalize these patterns and have not yet fully internalized the parental controls. Their behavior is normally tuned to the rewards and punishments that arise from the environment and not from within.

Middle Childhood

As the child grows to school age, longer periods of genuine sadness have been observed. These children are clearly unhappy although they are usually unable to give reasons for their plight. As this age, the child simply responds to his surroundings without much thought about who he is or how good or bad he is. Being good is what brings external reward and being bad is whatever provokes external punishment (Piaget, 1932). The child cannot form a stable sense of self in terms of worth and quite appropriately confuses fantasy with reality in his thoughts about himself. He does not have the capacity to sustain a consistent and continued low estimation of himself if any true estimation of self is indeed possible. Nevertheless, depreciation from others can adversely affect the child's mood. As Anna Freud (1970) remarked:

> Neurotic symptom formation waits until the ego has divided itself off from the id, but does not need to wait until ego and superego also have become two independent agencies. The

> first id-ego conflicts, and with them the first neurotic symptoms as conflict solutions, are produced with the ego under pressure from the environment, i.e., threatened not by guilt feelings arising internally from the superego but by dangers arising from the object world such as loss of love, rejection, punishment (p. 25).

Therefore the child can easily react with sadness to a chronically depriving environment or to an acute loss of needed sources of gratification. He may appear sad but this does not automatically imply an internal conflict. However, reports of such children (Sandler and Joffe, 1965; Poznanski and Zrull, 1970) do report some evidence of a cognitive transformation toward depression; these children are described as expecting bad treatment from others. Although they do not demean themselves, these children can generalize from their past frustrations with their parents to an intuitive attitude toward the rest of humanity.

Another reported finding is a tendency to give up when disappointed, which sets up a future predisposition toward hopelessness and helplessness after a blow to one's sense of self. It may well be that this early form of resignation results from accumulated experiences in which mastery was prevented and failure was insured by the responses of significant others. Therefore rejection or inflated, unrealistic demands by parents can lead to a sense that the child cannot win, that trying makes no sense. These findings tend to support Seligman's (1975) "learned helplessness" model as the root of depression. However, the actual situation is not so clear-cut. What seems to occur is that the parents reward certain behavior and show love, but only for activities that undermine the child's individuation and self-gratification. At this age the child's sense of worth is normally dependent on the responses of parental figures, so that their disapproval or rejection will have devastating effects and will inhibit the behavior that brought disapproval. As Sandler and Joffe remark, "It not infrequently happens that the child's parents are in unconscious opposition to progressive individuation, and the influence of the parents may be perpetuated in their successor, the superego" (1965, p. 54). At this age the child has not internalized a view of himself or a set of prohibitions, but he begins to automatically inhibit those behaviors that threaten to cut off the needed flow of approval from the parents.

We can perhaps define two types of dysphoric states in children of this age—one in which the parents gradually inhibit responses that would yield a sense of satisfaction or pleasure, and another in which the child directly responds to the deprivation of gratification in his environment. The former type can be seen in families in which the parents set up unrealistic ideals, use shame as a form of punishment, and are threatened by the child's individuation. The latter type is seen in homes where the parents are consistently rejecting or where they are themselves depressed. However, such dysphoric states frequently can be observed in children who are physically ill and whose illness interrupts their normal, everyday enjoyable activities.

The most extreme illustration of this latter form of dysphoria is a six-year-old boy reported by Bierman, Silverstein, and Finesinger (1958). This child had been hospitalized because of poliomyelitis. After two months of illness he manifested symptoms reminiscent of adult depression. He seemed to give up hope and lapse into a depressionlike withdrawal as he experienced day after day of frustration, confinement, and inability to participate in his usual gratifying activities. However, there is no record of self-recriminations, feelings of guilt, or low self-esteem. He was simply very unhappy at having lost the use of his legs. This was a true loss of enormous magnitude, and the child's response seems completely understandable and appropriate. His mother visited him regularly but her presence was insufficient in relieving the child's quite realistic sense of chronic deprivation. With clinical recovery of the primary illness, his mood returned to normal. This case is instructive since it demonstrates that children of this age are capable of extreme

sadness under chronically frustrating circumstances, but these moods are reactive to the environment and the child does not perpetuate a depressive mood in the absence of an external cause. However, one need not go to the extreme of a crippling illness and prolonged hospitalization to produce these moods; a chaotic family or a disapproving parent usually suffices.

Even in such instances the sadness is relatively short-lived. This short duration may be due to two major underlying characteristics of children of this age group: they are still creatures of the moment, and they will readily defend themselves against unpleasant feelings. The latter trait may account for conditions described as "depressive equivalents" or "masked depression" in children. Feelings of sadness often are defended against purely by distraction. The child simply attends to other more pleasant matters rather than to the environmental conditions that are causing him pain. If his attention is focused on these conditions, he will display the appropriate affect. However, this does not prove that an underlying or unconscious depression was present all along, seething beneath a seemingly happy exterior. The child maintains an amazing capacity to forget about tilings when not confronted by them. When this trait is coupled with normal childhood hedonism, it becomes clear why depressionlike symptoms should be rare and fleeting in this age group. It is only when the behavior appears to be excessive in its denial of an everpresent frustrating reality or the behavior is extremely maladaptive, that one should suspect a pathologic defensive denial of unpleasant affects, similar to what is seen in some adult hysterics.

The problem of "depressive equivalents" is more complex and at times confusing. Toolan (1962) lists eating and sleeping disorders, colic, and head-banging as depressive equivalents in infants, and temper tantrums, truancy, running away from home, and accident proneness as similar states in older children. Sperling (1959) suggests that sleep and gastrointestinal disorders in children may be equivalent to depression. These authors speculate that children cannot express depressive affect in an adult form, and these symptoms represent a childhood form of the disorder. This concept of symptom expression is clearly different from the "masked depression" described by Cytryn and McKnew (1972), who emphasize it as a childhood form of defense against feelings of depression.

Rie (1966) has written a thoughtful and thorough critique of the concepts of depressive equivalents in children. Briefly, Rie's major arguments are that: (1) There is no logical connection between the equivalent symptom and the alleged underlying depression. (2) There is no proof that any feeling of depression exists for which the symptom is taken as an equivalent. (3) Depression is inferred on the basis of theory only, so that any child who does not manifest depression directly after a loss must be expressing this painful affect in some other form. (4) Any symptom that can be interpreted as symbolic of oral deprivation (i.e., an eating disorder) has been mistakenly termed a psychodynamic equivalent to depression. Once again clinicians have projected their own expected reactions onto the psyche of a cognitively immature organism. Rather than assuming that depression must be present but expressed differently from adults, the possibility of the experience of adult forms of depression in a young child should be investigated more rigorously. This "adultomorphic" distortion perhaps has been utilized more in the stud}' of childhood depression than in any other pediatric psychiatric problem. The concept of depressive equivalents has done much to confuse the diagnostic status of childhood depression by allowing almost any symptom to be so classified. Until we know more about the inner life of children, it might be best to refrain from using this questionable concept.

In summary, children of early school age do display periods of prolonged unhappiness in response to chronic environmental stress. They are increasingly sensitive to the rejection of others as well as to deprivation of gratifications. However, these moods are rarely sustained and respond readily to external changes. Even in these states of sadness, there is no evidence of guilt or lowered self-regard. What may be present is an abnormal pressure to make the parent happy or to thwart personal satisfaction to obtain favor with the parent.

Late Childhood

At this stage of development, the child's cognitive abilities appear to allow for a system of thought that includes the sense of responsibility toward others, the internalization of values and rules, and a budding sense of one's self. Children of this age are normally less concerned with their families and more with the judgments of peers and society. However, they carry within themselves and into the community the internalized family belief systems that have been learned from the parents. Depending on the particulars of this belief system, the child will face frustration in a variety of ways[15] and derive different coping mechanisms. It is at this age that Sandler and Joffe's (1965) theoretical differentiation between depression as a psychobiological response and a clinical illness may assume particular importance. Children of this age not only react to disappointment or the loss of well-being with an initial depressive affective reaction, but they may continue to evolve a more chronic depressionlike illness. At this time the consolidation of adaptive processes takes place, so that the child will respond to stress in a repeated and characteristic manner. One such response, described by Sandler and Joffe (1965) and others, is to capitulate in the face of frustration and to develop a sense of overwhelming loss, a feeling of personal impotence, and shame.

The cognitive growth of the preadolescent years also allows for a recognition of the self which can be morally evaluated. The child may believe himself to be unworthy or unsatisfactory in the face of life's demands. Therefore, reports of dysphoric states at this stage do mention lowered self-regard. For example, McConville et al. (1973) described a subgroup of depressed children from eight to ten years old who expressed fixed ideas of negative self-esteem. Similarly, Poznanski and Zrull (1970) observed that older depressed children expressed disappointment in themselves rather than simply reacting to an external unpleasant situation.

Much of the deprivation of this age group appears to result from the child's thinking about his predicament and arriving at certain conclusions. The affect state is not an automatic consequence of experience, as in younger children; rather, it is a personal logical evaluation of the experience. Children of this age who cannot attain the parental ideal become depressed because they perceive this circumstance to be a personal failure and not simply that the parents are themselves unhappy. Similarly, older, repeatedly rejected children are reacting to their own belief that they are unlovable rather than only to the immediate pain of the rejection. Therefore, depression at this stage takes on a more cognitive, evaluative characteristic and in this sense is no longer the immediate, stimulus-bound sadness of the younger child. The younger child might directly seek dependency gratification or openly regress to infantile needs in the face of frustration, but these preadolescent children inhibit expression of these desires of which—like the adult—they feel ashamed. Behavior is scrutinized and evaluated in terms of the self. This cognitive aspect causes older children to remain depressed regardless of changes in external circumstances. Because of these selfperpetuating and self-evaluative aspects of the child's dysphoria, it may be correct to speak of actual depressive illness at this age. The point is that the depression results from cognitive conclusions which may be erroneous but are one step removed from the immediate environment.

Anthony and Scott (1960) reported a twelve-year-old child who manifested a depressive episode which may illustrate some of the features of depression in late childhood arising from pathological needs. Although this child's symptoms were much more severe than normally seen at this age, the underlying psychodynamics are not uncommon. This boy developed a severe depressive illness with manic interludes after his parents decided to adopt a ten-year-old boy to act as his companion. The patient suffered neither the loss of a love object nor the loss of gratifying activities, but was described as succumbing to depression as a result of the imagined loss of his favored status with his mother. His premorbid history was significant in many aspects: he was always overly close to his mother, he was timid and selfconscious, he rarely played with peers, he was unhappy at school (although he did well academically), and he generally solved his problems by giving up or by running to his mother. The authors described this patient as deriving a sense of omnipotence from being the "only fruit" of his mother's womb and the most precious thing in her world. The thought of sharing his mother with another child meant the loss of his inappropriate sense of self-meaning and an end to his pathological tie with her.

This child clearly suffered a depressive illness not only on the basis of his symptoms, but because his reaction was not in concert with the realistic stress; it evolved from his own distortions of the situation. His need for his mother was so great, and he had been so prevented from normal individuation and deprived of self-reliant sources of meaning and gratification, that at age twelve the prospect of another child entering the charmed mother-son circle was sufficient to cause a depressive decompensation.

Even in children who are this cognitively mature, however, the depression is not the same as in adults. The older child's self-evaluation is still more malleable than the adult's and more readily responds to positive environmental experiences. The negative sense of self is not so crystallized as to automatically devalue all successes or shun all gratifications. However, the major difference between depression at this stage and the adult variant is a lack of future orientation. The child during latency cannot truly relate his present state on a continuum with his future experience. Rather than denying the future defensively, he simply does not think of it. Rie (1966) made the pertinent observation that one of the crucial differences between adult and child depression may be the absence of hopelessness in the latter. Rie cited numerous definitions of adult depression and stressed that they all contain some reference to a time perspective that includes a representation of the future. He further argued that if the individual before adolescence cannot comprehend concepts such as long-range goals and their relationship to present strivings, the meaning of infinity, and the absolute permanence of loss or disappointment, then such an individual could not experience hopelessness and despair, two cardinal features of adult depression.[16]

Rie's arguments appear to be theoretically sound since Piaget (1952) also concluded that until early adolescence the child is wedded to the "concrete" and not capable of abstractions that would be involved in projecting himself into the future. Rie's conclusions also concur with clinical observations. Children do not complain of being unable to face tomorrow or that they will remain eternally depressed. They do not deny the prospect of an unbearable future; they simply do not think of it.

Adolescence

It is not until the end of childhood that depressive episodes truly comparable to adult states are seen clinically. The depressions of adolescence equal the adult forms in severity, surpass them in self-destructiveness, and still betray a characteristic developmental stamp. As mentioned before, the child does not appear able to conceive of his future; however, the adolescent seems capable of little else. The concept of time looms large is adolescent thought and in adolescent depression. There is the terrifying sense that all actions or experiences are irrevocable and everlasting, and result in eternal shame and despair. This overemphasis on the relationship of today with tomorrow is beyond the capacities of the child and is usually tempered by a greater life experience in the adult. For the adolescent, however, all seems lost and nothing can be redeemed.

Erikson (1959) has examined this distorted sense of time in his studies of disturbed adolescents who, from a different vantage point, can be seen as experiencing severe depressive episodes. Erikson notes: "Protests of a missed greatness and a premature and fatal loss of useful potential are common complaints among our patients as they are among adolescents in cultures which consider such protestations romantic; the implied malignancy, however, consists of a decided disbelief in the possibility that time may bring change, and yet also a fear that it might" (1959, p. 26). This fear of time and the inability to handle time appear to give adolescent depression an urgent, overwhelming quality.

Another factor that influences the expression of dysphoria in adolescence is the lack of moderation in thought. The adolescent appears to live in an all or nothing world; he gives seemingly unimportant events an inflated status and responds to them in a dramatic, allconsuming manner. Here again, the adolescent appears to lack sufficient maturity to put everyday events in proper perspective. Everything has an air of finality and, at times, of desperation.

Perhaps these attributes of adolescence are magnified by the social pressures that are exerted at this developmental phase in our own culture. I11 our society, youngsters are constantly reminded that they are building for their future lives—whether it is in terms of career, marriage, or social acceptance. This is also the age when many individuals are away from home for the first time, feeling unprepared for this responsibility and yet ashamed of what they perceive to be childish, dependent strivings. Such adolescents are so accustomed to living out the dictates of another that the availability of freedom leads to self-doubt and utter loneliness. They often form a tie with a new authority on whom they can depend for direction and meaning.

Other adolescents carry with them the need to reach some parental ideal only to find that either they are not able to reach it or to do so would mean giving up their own chance for individuation. Anthony (1975) uses John Stuart Mill's early difficulties to exemplify some pertinent aspects of depression in adolescence. Anthony writes that one day young Mill asked himself the crucial question: would he be happy if he accomplished all that his father had asked?

Mill was forced to answer no, and of that moment Mill wrote, "At this, my heart sank in me; the whole foundation on which my life was constructed fell down ... I seemed to have nothing to live for." Anthony explains "he fell ill when he became aware that the realization of his father's aims in life would not satisfy him, and he regained his mental health (to the degree that this was possible) when he understood that the death of the father brought with it the growth of identity, autonomy, and responsibility for the son" (1975, p. 448).

Not all adolescents are as fortunate as young Mill. Many continue to strive for the parental ideal which has become their ideal, denying life and pleasure and ultimately succumbing to depression whether or not the goal is ever reached. In adolescence one may observe the shaping of the characteristic forms of depression: the need for others, the dominant goal, and especially the ascetic self-denial that gradually erodes any experience of pleasure or meaning.

Conclusion

The foregoing sections have attempted to

apply a developmental approach to depressive phenomena in childhood. If depression is conceived of as a sophisticated affective experience that necessitates extensive cognitive maturation, then the dysphoric states that precede the experience of depression may be seen as continuous with, but not equal to, depression. The deprivation of the infant, the inhibition of the toddler, the stimulus-bound sadness of the young child, the limited depression of the older child, and the exaggerated yet acutely felt despair of the adolescent may all be understood best against a framework of the developmental process.

The types of reaction, the causes for their manifestation, and the underlying structural elements are presented in Table 8-1 with a parallel schema of ego development adapted from Loevinger (1976). Although obviously incomplete, such an attempt at synthesis may help in delineating the causes and types of depressionlike experience in childhood.

Table 8-1

Symptoms and Causes of Depression at Various Stages of Development

Developmental Stage	Symptoms	Major Psychodynamics
Infancy	Withdrawal after crying and protest	Loss of stimulation, security, and well being supplied by the mother
Early childhood	Inhibition, clinging behavior	Disapproval by parents
	Sadness as automatically responsive to the immediate situation	Rejection by parents, loss of gratifying activities (i.e., chronic illness)
		Unable to meet parental ideal, unable to sustain threat to parental relationship
	Depression with exaggerated urgency, time distortion, and impulsivity	Unable to fulfill internalized parental ideal, inability to separate from family.

Type of Dysphoria   Loevinger Ego Development Stages[17]

Deprivation of needed stimulation	Presocial, symbiotic
	Impulsive, self-protective, fear of being caught, externalizing blame, opportunistic
Sadness, unsustained crying directly related to frustrating or depriving situation	Conformist: conformity to external rules, shame and guilt for breaking rules, superficial niceness
Depression with a cognitive component in terms of affect resulting from deduction about circumstances	Conscientious: conformist, differentiation of norms and goals, awareness of self in relation to group, helping
Accentuation of depression by cognitive distortions about the finality of events	Conscientious: self-evaluated standards, guilt for consequences, longterm goals and ideals

Suicide in Children and Adolescents

Attempted or completed suicide in children appears to differ markedly from the selfdestructive behavior of adults. There are differences in frequency, sex distribution, effect of socio-cultural upheavals, and most significantly, in the motives underlying suicide in adults and children. As will be discussed further, there is some question whether the selfdestructive behavior of young children can be considered truly suicidal since they may have little appreciation of the meaning of death. There is even more question about a uniform association of suicide and depression in childhood. However, a sufficient number of depressed children and adolescents ultimately attempt suicide so that this topic may be considered here.

Statistical Data

Demographic reports (Seiden, 1969) suggest that the rate of suicide for children under fifteen years of age has changed little in this century. The general rate of 0.5 deaths per 100,000 population (for children under fifteen) (Seiden 1969) seems to have remained stable since 1900. This rate was unaffected by both World Wars (which decreased the total suicide rate) and by the Great Depression (which increased the total suicide rate). However, it is notoriously difficult to determine accurately the true rate of suicide in young children since such deaths may be greatly underreported. The suicides of young children are obviously tinged with shame, guilt, and embarrassment for the survivors so that the true nature of the death is concealed. Also, children do not leave suicide notes and there is greater opportunity for their deaths to be termed accidental.

In those cases where suicide cannot be doubted as the cause of death, it has been found that males outnumber females in actual suicides (Shaffer, 1974) although females may threaten suicide or make suicidal gestures more frequently (Mattson et al., 1969). Cultural beliefs also greatly influence the rate of suicide, especially in adolescents and young adults. Catholic countries such as Ireland, where suicide is considered a sin, have a low rate. In countries such as Japan, where suicide is considered an honorable way to die, self-destruction is the most common cause of death for individuals under thirty (Seiden, 1969). There is also some debate over hidden suicides in ghetto youths or among American Indians. "Hidden suicide" refers to youngsters who do not literally kill themselves (which would be considered cowardly) but force others to kill them through acts of delinquency or bravado. Wolfgang (1959) studied the Philadelphia police records and found a high number of such victim-precipitated homicides among black youths. Finally, while suicide is very rare in young children, its incidence increases rapidly with age and it is among the leading causes of death in older adolescents and young adults. Seiden quotes the Vital Statistics of the United States as recording the following rate of suicide by age group per 100,000 population in 1964: age five to nine, 0.05; age ten to fourteen, 0.4; age fifteen to nineteen, 4.6; and age twenty to twenty-four, 10.8. We can glean from these figures that there is a dramatic rise in the suicide rate as children grow toward maturity.

Motivation

Any attempt to deal with the motives behind the suicidal behavior of children must consider their concept of death. As stated by Seiden, many children want to kill themselves but they do not wish to die. This paradoxical statement becomes clear if we understand that many children do not consider death to be irreversible or perceive suicide as a grave act. Seiden cites the work of Winn and Halla, who found that young children attach as much significance to stealing from their mother's purse as they do to threatening to kill themselves.

The gradual development of the child's concept of death was studied by Schilder and Wechsler (1934) and later by Nagy (1959). The former investigators found that the young child does not believe in death as a natural termination of life but sees it as an event which can be caused only by violence or illness. Young children also do not believe in their own selfdestruction. Death is seen as a temporary, reversible state.

On the basis of projective materials such as drawings, written compositions, and verbal responses to questions asked of 378 children, Nagy described the development of the concept of death in children. She delineated three conceptual stages: children under age five conceive of death as a temporary, reversible state in which the individual is still alive but deprived of action, as in sleep. Between the ages of five and nine, the child begins to appreciate death as a fearful state in which one is separated from loved ones. Death is personified as a "skeleton man" who carries off children at night, and is thought of as a fortuitous external event and not as a certain eventuality. Children at this stage also identify death with physical changes (i.e., a dead person is all bones) rather than with a possible obliteration or transformation of consciousness. Around age nine, children begin to exhibit an adult view of death as the termination of life and as universal. As one boy of nine years, 11 months put it, "Death is something that no one can escape."

Anthony (1967) postulated an "eight-year anxiety" in the child which consists of a preoccupation with ideas of death or dying, either about himself or his parents. In agreement with Nagy, he found that around this age the child realizes death is irreversible and also feels helpless in the face of its inevitability, since everyone is in the same predicament. This phase passes quickly and a sense of personal immunity soon reasserts itself. However, if traumatic events occur during this phase, there may be an additional challenge to the child's defenses and pathology may result.

On the basis of these studies, it is questionable if self-destructive acts before age nine or ten can be truly considered suicidal. In many cases, even after this age (and also in some adults) the individual appears to momentarily deny the extreme gravity of death in order to escape an intolerable situation or to punish others by a suicidal act. Such extreme measures, however, only can occur against a background of a lack of compassion and care. As to why very young children do not appear to kill themselves since they deny the permanence of death and are impulsive, a logical possibility is Shaffer's suggestion (1974) that they lack the cognitive maturity to carefully plan suicide or even the knowledge of how to carry out the act.

In rare instances in which a childhood death by suicide can be substantiated, researchers have found a few predominant themes which seem to underlie most of these acts. As early as 1855, Durand-Fardel reviewed all suicides by persons under sixteen years of age in France between 1835 and 1844. Of the 192 childhood suicides reported, he was able to study 22 such incidents in detail. Of these, ten children drowned themselves, ten hanged themselves, and two burned themselves. There is no mention of death by ingestion of toxic substances or by overdose of drugs, which today is the most prevalent form of self-destruction. However, the motives behind childhood suicide have remained essentially the same over a century. DurandFardel mentions fear of impending punishment, reproach for a misdeed, an attempt to punish the parents, or the wish to join a dead loved one as reasons for suicide. Overall, he makes an impassioned plea for better treatment of children. He also observes that it is the deprivation of love rather than material goods that predisposes childhood suicide: "In the poorhouse of farmers as well as in the houses of workers and educated people, one finds children that cannot take the absence of tenderness. They cannot cope with brutality and injustice."

Later studies have echoed these themes. Bender and Schilder in 1937 studied eighteen children under thirteen years of age who were admitted to the Bellevue psychiatric ward with manifested suicidal preoccupations. They found that these children came from backgrounds of emotional deprivation in which they did not receive the amount of love they desired or needed. This deprivation was said to arouse feelings of aggression against the parents but, because of concomitant guilt, the aggression was allegedly turned against the self, resulting in suicidal wishes. Bender and Schilder also noted other suicidal motives in their sample such as the children's wish to punish those around them, to attain the desired love by coercion, and to be reunited with a departed love object. Despert

(1952) came to similar conclusions fifteen years later, in studying a group of children who had unsuccessfully attempted suicide.

Shaffer (1974) recently investigated contemporaneous data on children who actually committed suicide. He reports detailed information on thirty-one children under the age of fifteen who killed themselves in England and Wales between the years 1962 and 1968. In over one-third of the cases, the precipitating event was a disciplinary crisis of some sort— usually the anticipation of punishment. Other precipitants in order of frequency were problems with peers, disputes with parents, being dropped from a school team, interaction with a psychotic parent, and imitation of a "fantasy model," meaning that the child was copying the act of a well-publicized suicide. The personality descriptions of these children were: (1) children who felt that others didn't like them, (2) children who were quiet and uncommunicative, and (3) children who were perfectionist and self-critical. The first of these descriptions overlapped with the others, and a fourth type of personality found in six cases, that of being impulsive and erratic, did not coincide at all. Shaffer concludes that suicidal children may conform to two stereotypes: children of superior intellect who were isolated from peers and possibly became depressed; and children who were impetuous, prone to aggressive outbursts, and overly sensitive to criticism. While such stereotypes may be familiar to psychiatric profiles, the propensity to suicide is believed to reside in their familiarity with the phenomenon of suicide itself. Shaffer backs up this supposition with the finding that the families of these children showed a high incidence of attempted suicide and depression (with possible talk of suicide).

Shaffer concludes that childhood suicide is the end result of many factors, not the least of which is a certain cognitive maturity both in terms of what death actually means and in terms of being able to plan and execute a suicidal plan. Other significant variables were a disturbed family background, a depressed mental state, a precipitating incident (often of a humiliating kind), access to a means of suicide, and close experience with suicidal behavior. Out of respect for the family's sensibilities, Shaffer did not directly interview the surviving family members and thus does not stress the emotional deprivation so strongly emphasized by other investigators.

The following case example may help in giving an idea of the familial atmosphere so often found in the evaluation of suicidal children.

Illustrative Case Study Of Suicidal Child

Donna was an eleven-year-old girl who told her teacher that she was planning to kill herself and had been contemplating suicide for some time. This "confession" did not appear to be a manipulative gesture but was divulged in the context of a personal talk with the teacher whom Donna preferred to her own mother. Donna was the oldest of four children and was expected to be responsible for her younger sibs. They would tease her but she could not retaliate for fear of being punished by her parents. Donna had been raped by a relative when she was six years old, and apparently had borne the brunt of blame for this incident. Her mother continually accused Donna of being promiscuous and of having secret liaisons with boys despite the fact that the girl was only eleven years of age. The mother kept a close watch over Donna and did not allow her any significant extrafamilial relationships. She had to be home directly after school and she frequently was beaten by both parents. One week prior to her "confession" to the teacher, Donna's mother in a fit of rage said she would kill her and Donna believed her. She decided it would be better to take her own life instead. When the mother was seen, she denied any history of child abuse (despite documented evidence to the contrary). It was learned that the father probably had had a series of affairs which infuriated the mother. Both parents seemed to utilize Donna as a scapegoat for their own frustrations. If she had not found some comforting outsider and revealed her plan, she may well have killed herself.

Suicidal Behavior In Adolescence

A totally different picture emerges when adolescent suicide is considered. Suicide among adolescents is not rare, and gestures or attempts are very frequent. Suicide ranks as a leading cause of death among the fifteen- to nineteenyear age group and 12 percent of all suicide attempts are made by teenagers (of these, 90 percent are female) (Seiden, 1969). The reasons for this high rate of self-destructive behavior are not completely understood. Some authors believe that depression is a significant predisposition and others believe anger toward others is the major determinant. Here again, semantics confuses the issue since some authors will classify depression only when there is clear evidence of anger turned toward the self, ignoring responses to loss or frustration and often labelling these latter states as grief reactions. Therefore the prevalence of depression among teenagers who attempt suicide remains largely a matter of how the particular author defines depression.

Mattson et al. (1969) distinguished six groups of child and adolescent suicide attempters in their study of seventy-five patients at a psychiatric clinic. The motivations for each group were: (1) Loss of a love object: these patients sustained the death or desertion of a parent or peer of the opposite sex. They were depressed and wished to die in order to join the deceased person. Although lonely and sad, they did not exhibit guilt or self-recriminations (three boys, fourteen girls). (2) "The bad me," that is, markedly self-depreciating patients: these patients hated themselves and felt they deserved to die. They viewed death as a solution and possible rebirth as a more worthy person (nine boys, eleven girls). (3) The final "cry for help" directed beyond the immediate family: these patients appeared worn out by chronic overwhelming external stress such as physical illness or family disruption (one boy, fourteen girls). (4) The revengeful, angry teenager: these adolescents clearly stated the coercive, manipulative aspects of their suicidal gestures and did not actually intend to kill themselves (three boys, ten girls). (5) The psychotic adolescent: these patients made repeated suicide threats, and suicide seemed to be a desperate solution to inner tension and confusion rather than an acting out of delusional belief (two boys, five girls). (6) "The suicide game": these patients flirted with death in order to get peer approval and to experience a thrill. They exhibited denial of death and questionable suicidal intent (one boy, two girls).

This breakdown of a large sample of suicidal children, mostly teenagers, demonstrates the variety of motivations for self-destructive behavior. It is significant that girls outnumbered boys over two to one in suicidal threats and gestures, while the actual suicides committed in the same geographic area for the same time period were all committed by adolescent boys using firearms.

From these and other data, it may be concluded that although adolescent girls more frequently attempt suicide, more adolescent boys actually kill themselves. The main feature which seems to differentiate true suicidal intent from suicidal gestures is social isolation (Seiden, 1969). As long as there is someone to whom the teenager can turn for help or against whom he can vent his rage, true suicide may be averted. If the youngster believes no one who will care if he lives or dies, then suicide becomes a real possibility. Many of the attempts or gestures may be seen as desperate communications to others, but true suicides are well planned with no chance of survival. Two difficulties that obviously attend gestures are that the attempt may misfire and the individual die unintentionally; or if this desperate gesture is not taken seriously by loved ones, the youngster may be convinced that no one really does care and then attempt a true suicidal act.

A subgroup which has received considerable attention is the suicidal college student. Students attending Harvard or Yale showed twice the suicide rate as nonstudents of the same age (Seiden, 1969). Similar findings were obtained from studying the suicide rates at

Oxford and Cambridge in England (cited in Seiden). Investigations of the differences between suicidal and nonsuicidal classmates revealed that the former group was older, did better academically, and showed more indications of emotional disturbance. There was also a greater number of foreign students among the suicidal group, which may indicate separation from the usual social support systems and a greater sense of isolation. Some authors have mentioned fear of academic failure, extreme scholastic pressure, or shame over feelings of inadequacy and dependency as major suicidal motives in the college student. Again, there is no uniform motivation that can account of all suicidal behavior. On the other hand, Hendin (1975) proposed some common characteristics among students who attempt suicide. He eloquently wrote that some individuals are drawn to death as a way of life: they are so inhibited and tied to a past familial atmosphere of gloom and despair that they cannot tolerate the opportunities for pleasure and involvement which college life offers them.

> These students see their relationships with their parents as dependent on their emotional if not physical death and become tied to their parents in a death knot. Coming to college, graduating, becoming seriously

> involved with another person, and enjoying an independent existence have the power to free them. In fact, the meaning of suicide and depression lies in their encounter with the forces that might unleash their own possibilities for freedom (pp. 238-239).

For such individuals, numbness is a sort of protection and the possibility of gratifications arouses guilt over betraying a secret bond with the parent. This guilt and the understanding that it blocks pleasure leaves the individual frozen in a state of inhibition; he cannot break through the old sanctions and yet cannot endure living in accordance with them. Suicide becomes a possible solution to this conflict. Death has always held a special fascination for these individuals who, according to Hendin, by their own self-destruction appear to fulfill the parental command not to dare to live.

Hendin's work draws attention to some of the potent forces for suicide in all age groups: a lack of being appreciated for what one is, a failure of parents to instill a sense of joy and approval of life in the child, and finally, a prevailing sense in the individual that his enjoyment of other relationships or other activities is a guilty betrayal. Suicide, like depression, may ultimately result from a selfinduced elimination of satisfactory and satisfying life alternatives that are not tied to omnipotent others or dominating goals. This lack of freedom to form new interests or relationships—that is, a lack of freedom to enjoy life—results in depression and ultimately in some suicides. If the adolescent can achieve some wholly personal aspect of life, free from the deadening burden of guilt and parental "shoulds," he may escape the premature termination of his own potential. Some adolescents find solace in a relationship, a cause, or an academic interest which may lead them to liberation and away from their heritage of obligation and self-denial.

In his autobiography Bertrand Russell recalls the cold and unloving atmosphere in which he grew up. Throughout his teens he often considered doing away with himself, but he survived to live a long and productive life. He wrote, looking back at the time he was fifteen, "There was a footpath leading across fields to New Southgate, and I used to go there alone to watch the sunset and contemplate suicide. I did not, however, commit suicide, because I wished to know more of mathematics" (1967, p. 45).

Notes

[15] The Freudian concept of the superego does not entirely do justice

Continued Understanding in Depression (Part 2)

to the internalized cognitive system. The superego seems to be limited to punishment and idealization while the internalized cognitive system assumes many of the functions normally ascribed to the ego, such as modes of adaptation, self-assessment, and relationships with others.

[16] Rie's argument is equally important for showing again how depression is ultimately dependent on the development of the capacities of the ego (especially cognitive abilities) rather than simply on the formation of the superego.

[17] Adapted from Loevinger, J. 1976. *Ego development.* San Francisco: Jossey-Bass.